A Drug-Free Appro...
to Asperger Syndrome
and Autism

Homeopathic Care for
Exceptional Kids

A Drug-Free Approach to Asperger Syndrome and Autism

Homeopathic Care for
Exceptional Kids

Judyth Reichenberg-Ullman, N.D., L.C.S.W.
Robert Ullman, N.D.
Ian Luepker, N.D.

Picnic Point Press

Published by: Picnic Point Press
                       131 Third Avenue North
                       Edmonds, WA 98020
                       (800) 398-1151

ISBN 0-9640654-6-0

1 2 3 4 5 6 / 09 08 07 06 05
Printed in the United States of America

To Order: Visit us online at
www.drugfreeasperger.com
or call: (800) 398-1151

*We dedicate this book to Angela
and to all others who follow their
grand passion with heart and in truth.*

Contents

Foreword

Homeopathy is becoming increasingly well-accepted in the United States, as it has been in Europe for many years. A major reason for the upsurge in the popularity of homeopathy is the rapidly diminishing respect for conventional, traditional, "establishment" medicine. The concept behind homeopathy contrasts sharply with the assumptions of conventional American medicine.

Homeopathy embodies the idea that many of the symptoms of disease are actually manifestations of the body's attempts to heal itself. The homeopathic doctor sees his or her role as facilitating these efforts of the body to heal itself by administering medicines or "remedies" which will stimulate and augment the symptoms. Conventional U.S. medicine, also known as allopathic medicine, takes the opposite view—it assumes that if you give drugs which fight the symptoms rather than enhance them, the disease will disappear. Both of these competing theories, homeopathy and allopathy, have a certain amount of plausibility. The debate between advocates and practitioners of both sides has gone on for centuries.

Why, in recent years, has homeopathy suddenly become ascendant at the expense of allopathy? There are no doubt many answers to that question, but in my opinion the most important of those reasons is that as medical recordkeeping has become more bureaucratized, computerized and more accurate, it has become increasingly apparent that allopathy's use of drugs carries with it a terrible penalty in terms of sickness, death and malpractice insurance costs. The pharmaceutical companies which manufacture the drugs used by allopathic physicians have become billion-dollar behemoths, perhaps the most profitable industry in the world. The pharmaceutical companies have more lobbyists in Washington, D.C. than there are congressmen and senators. Despite the hundreds of millions of dollars spent on lobbying, on public relations campaigns and on advertisements for various drugs, the public has been learning, especially in the past year or two, that prescription drugs are neither as beneficial as they are claimed to be, nor anywhere as safe as one would hope they should be. An estimated 160,000 people a year in the U.S. die as a result of adverse drug reactions, and several million are severely injured.

Elsewhere I have characterized traditional medicine —allopathy—as an attempt (a misguided attempt) to bring about health through the administration of sublethal doses of toxic substances. Strange, but true. All too often the doses turn out to be lethal rather than sublethal. I especially like the title of this book: *A Drug-Free Approach*. The allopathic drugs which are routinely used to treat autistic children can produce a horrific array of adverse reactions.

Homeopathy is rapidly rising in popularity for a number of reasons, which include: 1. Safety—serious adverse reactions, especially death, are virtually unheard of with the use of homeopathic remedies. 2. Homeopathy is far more cognizant of the individuality of the patient— it embraces the concept that there is no such entity as a disease, only an interaction between a disease process and an individual patient. 3. Homeopathy recognizes and appreciates the fact—and it is a fact—that the body is far better informed and far wiser than any or all of us.

Helping the body heal itself makes sense, in many ways.

The authors of this long-awaited book have a wealth of experience using the principles of homeopathy to treat patients on the autism spectrum. I am pleased indeed that they have elected to share their experiences with us by writing this book.

Bernard Rimland, Ph.D
Founder and Director
Autism Research Institute
San Diego, California

Acknowledgments

We respectfully thank Bernard Rimland, Ph.D., a pioneer in the field of autism, for taking time out of his busy schedule to write the foreword. The multi-talented Lynn Willeford produced an astute, and remarkably rapid, copy edit. We were fortunate to work with Ann Amberg, who did a great job on internal book design, typesetting, and indexing. We thank Pat Rasch for an eye-catching and compelling cover. We express our appreciation to Diane Twachtman-Cullen, Ph.D for her invaluable edit of our first draft. Our gratitude to Libby Urner, experienced editor, as well as mom of a son with AS, who has responded very favorably to homeopathy, for a generous first edit. Our special thanks to Jan Maxon, special education teacher, mother of two children whose cases appear in this book, and who is an ardent and vocal supporter of our work with children on the spectrum.

Above all, we cannot praise highly enough, our remarkable office staff—Tracy Huntsman, Krystyne Kenney, and Jeanie Blair—without whose help we never could have treated these children, and who have offered ongoing help and encouragement to their parents and to us. They also make our office a great place to work and a lot of fun! Lastly, we offer biscuits to our golden retriever mascots, Chai and Truffle, who shower us, our staff, and our patients with gentle affection and unconditional love.

Introduction

Holding Hope for a Better Answer
to Help Your Child with ASD

If you are a parent of a child with Asperger Syndrome (AS) or some other autism spectrum disorder (ASD), you have probably read enough books on the subject to fill a small library. You may have visited countless web sites, chatted personally or online with dozens of supportive parents, and tried more diets, supplements, various therapies and medications than you could have imagined. You may know more about ASD and related diagnoses than many doctors. The myriad of abbreviations—ASD, AS, ADHD, OCD, ODD, SPD, BPD, and so on (see Glossary)—may seem like an endless array of labels, none of which adequately fits your child. Perhaps you have grown tired of experimenting with one pharmaceutical drug after another, including stimulants, anti-depressants, anti-anxiety medications, anticonvulsants, and antipsychotics. Perhaps you found them to be either ineffective for treating the core symptoms of ASD or rife with unwanted side effects. Or you may simply not feel comfortable giving your child psychiatric medications.

But, you continue to hold hope for a better answer, or you would not even be picking up this book. You cling fiercely to the conviction that there must be a way to find help for your child. You want the very best for your child—for him to reach his highest potential and happiness. You hold a vision of the fulfillment of your child's dreams and aspirations; and you are determined to leave no stone unturned when it comes to your child's healing and well being.

If You're Looking For a Drug-Free Approach to ASD, Read This Book!

There are many different approaches for children on the autism spectrum. You may be wondering, what makes this book different from all the others you've read? We offer an approach that is natural, safe, and free of side effects that can offer significant, even dramatic, results for children with ASD and other developmental, behavioral, and learning problems. Let us share with you what we have found in our work with these remarkable patients. After you read about the children we have been able to help using homeopathic medicine, you may find it to be an avenue you wish to pursue further.

What if we told you about an approach to treating ASD that was individualized, addressed all of your child's problems at once, looked at your child as a unique person rather than a diagnosis, and could be used along with conventional medicine, or even replace it? And what if the medicines tasted so good that kids begged for more?

If you're an open-minded, curious type of person, we hope we have stirred your curiosity. If you're a diehard skeptic, these claims may seem implausible, if not impossible. But they are not. The cases in this book are those of real patients from our practice (identities have been disguised for privacy). Even if you have never even heard of homeopathy, if you have any interest in the subject of ASD we believe you will find this book intriguing and, quite possibly, a lifesaver.

Who Are We to Be Talking About ASD?

We, Dr. Reichenberg-Ullman and Dr. Ullman, are licensed naturopathic physicians board-certified in homeopathic medicine in practice for over twenty years. Dr. Luepker joined our practice as a naturopathic physician in 2002, works with us closely as an associate, and has obtained his board certification in homeopathic medicine. Each of us had extensive psychiatric training and experience prior to attending naturopathic medical school, and we have a special interest in helping patients with mental and emotional problems.

Seventeen years ago, a patient who cared for seriously disturbed foster children started bringing her charges to us for homeopathic care. We witnessed such impressive changes in many of these children, not just physically, but emotionally, mentally, and behaviorally, that we started presenting these cases, respecting confidentiality, to the public. Case conferences and articles in publications such as *Mothering* magazine resulted in our treating a growing number of children with Attention Deficit Hyperactivity Disorder (ADHD) and other behavioral and learning problems. This led to our writing the bestselling *Ritalin-Free Kids*, which struck a chord with many parents seeking a natural alternative to drugs.

Since then we have treated over 4,000 children from all over the United States and beyond, not only for ADHD, but for a wide range of other problems and diagnoses. Given the precipitous rise in the number of children diagnosed with ASD, it is no surprise that we are seeing a growing number of these youngsters in our practice. Since so many children with ASD are initially diagnosed with ADHD, we recognize a number of former patients who would also likely be diagnosed today with ASD.

Our First Patient With ASD

Zachary, our first ASD patient, came to us over twelve years ago at the age of four and a half. This child was a long-awaited blessing from heaven, an only child born to parents already married sixteen years. A shy little boy with a wiry, delicate frame, Zach had a number of traits that we now recognize to be typical of kids with ASD.

What first caught our attention was Zach's habit of scrunching up his face into a curious grimace. He also had the habit of talking to himself repetitively, echoing back whatever his mom said, and counting aloud in whispers. He was a bright boy though, and by the age of two years and three months Zachary had learned the alphabet and numbers up to fifty and had begun to read. By the time he reached preschool, he was two years ahead of his peers. An extraordinarily picky eater, Zach steadfastly refused to venture a bite of any food that was the least bit unfamiliar.

A highly sensitive boy, Zach withdrew from conflicts and felt uncomfortable around strangers. Most cartoons were far too violent for his taste. Touch was another area in which Zach's sensitivities were hyper-acute. Whenever his hair was touched, he let out a scream. He was loath to touch even a plantain flower because of its spikiness. When exposed to loud noises, the child would cover his ears and grimace, as if in terrible pain. So low was Zach's pain threshold that even minor scrapes that would go unnoticed by other children caused him extreme suffering. The tiniest bug and spider bites resulted in large, open sores.

It was Zachary's sleep problems that led his mom to bring him to us. Shortly after his fourth birthday, he began to awaken around midnight, and then again at 4:00 a.m., agitated and fearful. The sound of the wind and the noise of cars on the highway made it impossible for the child to sleep soundly. In turn, Zach's restless sleep patterns disrupted his parents' rest, since he reported promptly to their bedroom each time he awoke.

Strange, Rare, and Peculiar

In treating children like Zachary, homeopaths are trained to zero in on anything unusual or unexpected about an individual. In the homeopathic literature, such symptoms are called *strange, rare, and peculiar.* The homeopathic approach is the opposite of the conventional medical approach of pigeon-holing individuals into diagnostic categories. Homeopaths listen carefully for what we have not heard before in order to discover what makes that person different from everyone else, even those with the same diagnosis.

In Zachary's case, we were struck by his exaggerated reaction to a level of noise that would be tolerable to the average child. Though Zach had a variety of somewhat odd characteristics, this sensitivity to noise was the most extreme. We gave him one dose of *Theridion*, a homeopathic medicine made from a small West Indian spider found on orange trees. It is well indicated for children who, among other symptoms, experience over-sensitivity to, or fear of, noise.

When Zach's mom brought him back to see us two and a half months later, she was very pleased. Noticeably less anxious, Zach was sleeping much more restfully. His sensitivities had settled down considerably, though he still covered his ears when confronted by loud noises. The grimacing and self-talk were gone. Over the next year and a half, Zach continued to improve steadily. The night waking, grimacing, and self-talk did not return. His sensitivity to noise was dramatically reduced.

We didn't hear again from Zachary until three years ago, when his mother brought him back in for situational depression and hay fever. Because the majority of his ASD symptoms had resolved, Zach's mom had seen no reason to continue homeopathic treatment during the intervening period of time. This time his hay fever resolved within days of taking *Sabadilla* (Mexican cevadilla), and the depression improved significantly within several weeks. After eight months, his mother again discontinued treatment. The last time we had any information about Zach was a report a year ago from his mom, who referred to her son as a "normal teenager".

Since treating Zach, we have had the opportunity to treat a growing number of youngsters on the autism spectrum, often with gratifying results. Homeopathy cannot help every child, but when treatment is successful, the outcome is well worth the investment of time and money. The parents of the children whose cases appear in this book are very glad that they took the leap to try homeopathic medicine.

Why Homeopathy Is a Particularly Good Fit for Children With ASD

Homeopaths are detectives. We often use the analogy of a jigsaw puzzle to describe the process of finding the homeopathic medicine that best matches a person's symptoms. Imagine that your child's symptoms were the scattered fragments of a three-hundred-piece puzzle. At first glance, the pieces would appear unrelated to each other and would not form a recognizable pattern. The goal is to correctly assemble all of the separate pieces into an identifiable image. First, you need to select those pieces that obviously fit together to make up at least a portion of a distinguishable image. Say, for example, it was a puzzle of the Statue of Liberty. If you found a torch or a crown and noticed that most of the pieces were green, you would have sufficient clues to recognize the structure and to be certain that it was not the Eiffel Tower. The Manhattan skyline in the background would confirm even further that it was the Statue of Liberty.

The same is true when a homeopath treats a child. Our goal is to recognize enough pieces of the puzzle of who your child is to suggest one particular homeopathic medicine. The more unique the features of the child, the easier it is to find the medicine that is likely to produce a positive response.

In the case of a child with ASD, we typically find a wealth of individualizing characteristics such as idiosyncratic habits, behaviors, mannerisms, and quirks, to narrow down the choice of possible medicines to one or several among over 2,000 possibilities. It is those very features that make a child with ASD stand out from *neurotypical* (NT) children that are the keys to his successful homeopathic treatment.

A Medicine Whose Time Has Come

Conventional medicine cannot yet provide a conclusive answer as to why so many children are being diagnosed with autism spectrum disorders, much less offer a cure. Since an increasing number of parents feel their needs are not being met by mainstream medicine, we invite you to take a good look at another approach—one that treats people, not diagnoses. Homeopathic medicine has been around over two hundred years, is widely practiced worldwide, and is safe even for pregnant mothers, newborns, young children, and the elderly.

Homeopathy holds the possibility of helping your child significantly, so that he can become all that he can be and can enjoy the health, happiness, and opportunities he deserves.

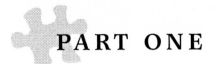

PART ONE

Homeopathy:
A Drug-Free Approach
to Asperger Syndrome

1

Strangers in a Strange Land
Core Features of Asperger Syndrome

Children and adults with Asperger Syndrome often feel like Valentine Michael Smith, the main character in Robert Heinlein's classic science-fiction novel, *Stranger in a Strange Land*. The last human survivor of a failed expedition to Mars, and raised from infancy by Martians, Smith possesses superior intelligence, but has the social and communication skills of an alien toddler. The excerpt below gives some indications of the challenges he faces soon after returning to Earth as a twenty-five year-old adult.

> *None of his thinkings [sic] had been in Earth symbols. Simple English he had freshly learned to speak, but much less easily than a Hindu uses it to trade with a Turk. Smith used English as one might use a code book, with tedious and imperfect translation for each symbol. Now his thoughts, pure Martian abstractions from half a million years of wildly alien culture, traveled so far from any human experience as to be utterly untranslatable... He looked the room over, noting without discrimination and with praise all of its details, both unimportant and important. He was in fact seeing it for the first time, as he had been incapable of enfolding it when he had been brought there the day before. The commonplace*

room was not commonplace to him, there was nothing remotely like it on Mars.[1]

For Valentine Michael Smith, and for those with Asperger Syndrome (AS), the world may seem an incomprehensible place, an alien planet where one is held against one's will, without even a guidebook. (Throughout this book we will use AS to denote this high functioning form of autism and ASD to denote Autism Spectrum Disorder, an "umbrella" term indicating the wider spectrum of autistic disorders.) Imagine what it is like to be highly intelligent, but to continually misunderstand facial expressions, gestures, and social cues. Imagine further what it is like to miss out on the subtle nuances in communication that are so fundamental to expressing humor, sarcasm, irritation, or sympathy, while those closest to you throw up their hands in exasperation at decisions that seem completely logical to you. This is the plight of the AS child or adult. Imagine how challenging it would be to live this way for one day, for even one hour, without becoming confused, depressed, anxious, frustrated, or angry. People with AS populate this alien world every day, day after day. Adapting to the social world depends on their learning effective communication and social skills, understanding how differently those around them think and reason, and expressing feelings that don't always make sense.

Again, Valentine Michael Smith's plight in *Stranger in a Strange Land* brings this lack of comprehension, and the resultant frustration, alive:

Doctor Archer Frame...walked in at that moment. "Good morning," he said. "How do you feel?" Smith turned the question over in his mind. The first phrase he recognized as a formal sound, requiring no answer, but which could be repeated or might not be. The second phrase was listed in his mind with several possible translations...He felt that dismay which so often overtook him in trying to communicate with these creatures, a frightening sensation, unknown to him before he met men. But he forced his body to remain calm and risked an answer. "Feel good."

"Good," the creature echoed. "Doctor Nelson will be along in a minute. Feel like some breakfast?"

All four symbols were in Smith's vocabulary, but he had trouble believing he had heard them rightly. He knew that he was food, but he did not feel like food. Nor had he had any warning that he might be selected for such an honor. He had not known the food supply was such that it was necessary to reduce the corporate group. He was filled with mild regret, since there was still so much to grok [understand deeply] of these new events.[2]

Smith, using his Martian frame of reference, interpreted what he was hearing literally, taking a simple colloquial inquiry about whether he wanted breakfast to potentially mean he had been selected as a food sacrifice for the sake of the group! An individual with AS, given the circumstances, might consider Smith's line of reasoning perfectly logical. Wired differently from their neurotypical (NT) peers, relationships between those with AS and their NT peers can flounder in a bewildering mix of missed communications, mismatched thought processes, and diametrically different assumptions about the world and life.

AS: the Evolution of a Diagnosis

In 1944, a Viennese pediatrician named Hans Asperger described four patients who, despite adequate verbal and cognitive intelligence, demonstrated problems with social interaction, communication, and idiosyncratic interests. He originally used the term *autistic psychopathy* to characterize these patients. Much of what Dr. Asperger observed in Vienna during the 1930s has been incorporated into the current diagnostic description of Asperger Syndrome. His observations are as relevant today as they were seventy years ago.

The term Asperger Syndrome was coined in a 1981 paper by Lorna Wing, and has since come into common usage for describing a type of Autism Spectrum Disorder (ASD) or Pervasive Developmental Disorder (PDD). Over the next decade, case reports and research steadily increased, until AS was officially categorized in the tenth edition of the International Classification of Diseases (ICD-10), published in 1993. A year later, the Diagnostic and Statistical Manual of Mental Disorders (DSM-IV) officially included AS.

Even with today's diagnostic criteria, describing AS is challenging because no two cases are alike, even within the same family. Despite this, recognizable, shared features can be identified. These traits and characteristics can point, at least roughly, to who fits within the diagnostic criteria. Below, we have described some of the core traits of AS. Many of the following thirteen hallmarks may be very familiar to you.

- Blindness to social cues
- Problems communicating
- Apparent lack of empathy
- Minimal eye contact

- Restricted repertoire of interests
- Need for structure and routine
- Trouble fitting in
- Literal to a fault
- Bizarre behaviors
- Difficulties with sports
- Precocious reading ability
- Physical hypersensitivity
- Fear of failure and low self-esteem

The Core Characteristics of AS

Blindness to social cues

To a child with AS, the world of people and social interaction may seem fuzzy and out of focus. A great deal of
communication occurs nonverbally through facial expression, eye contact, gesture, and body language. Someone
with AS may misunderstand—or miss entirely—social
cues, facial expressions, and motivations. In some con-
texts, nonverbal communication speaks even louder than
words. What if you were in Rome, having just learned
Italian in a six-week crash course. You might be able to
understand most of the words you hear individually, but
could still have difficulty fitting them into meaningful
sentences. The use of slang and idiom would probably be
completely confusing. To make things worse, the hand
gestures and body motions of the Italians might seem so
varied and intense, that you could only understand a
small portion of what was actually being conveyed. For
example, you might innocently think that the large man
patting his bicep forcefully while raising his right arm in
your direction wants to demonstrate how strong he is
when in fact, he is making an extremely obscene and disrespectful gesture.

This example is analogous to the state of the child with AS, who not only may have difficulty with understanding verbal communication, but often hasn't a clue when it comes to gestures, facial expressions, and body language. A child with AS shown photographs of people with facial expressions that any NT child could easily identify might be at a loss to explain which ones depict happiness and which depict sadness, anger or fear.[3]

Considerable training and practice may be necessary before a child with AS can even begin to read facial expressions in real-life situations. More complex forms of gesture and body language, or the combination of these with known facial expressions, may be even more difficult to grasp. A mother who is looking angry, speaking loudly, and shaking her index finger may have little impact on a child with AS, who may not alter his behavior in response to such a display because he does not understand its meaning. The mother, puzzled, may use a louder tone or more forceful gestures, further confusing the child, who still is not getting the message that is so clear to the mom.

Problems communicating

Children with AS struggle with communication, and their speech maybe distinctly odd. While their vocabulary development may be far beyond their years, using words correctly in spontaneous conversation or communicating within a social context may be a problem.

Conversation is typically one-sided, more monologue than dialogue, and often revolves around one all-encompassing, repetitive topic. Children with AS tend to unilaterally dominate conversations, interfering with the usual give and take of two-way conversation. Their memory for facts and details can seem astonishing, even mesmerizing, at first. The novelty soon wears off when the one-sided nature of the interaction becomes evident. Unless the listener is family, or is socially obligated to engage in conversation, he may look for the nearest exit, and leave the youngster at the first opportunity. While adults may put up with this kind of monologue for a while, children may have no patience for it, and quickly lose interest. This is one reason why kids with AS gravitate to adults rather than to peers. Even if the special interest is peer-appropriate, such as Harry Potter or GameBoy, the level of detail and monopolizing often lead to frustration and an expression of "enough is enough" or "can't you talk about something else?"

The pragmatics of language (the practical use of language in a social setting) doesn't come easily to a child with AS. For instance, a child may start a conversation with a completely irrelevant and untimely comment, such as asking a stranger, immediately before a church service begins, if he is familiar with the straight-six, 200-horsepower engine used in the 1966 Ford Mustang. As the service commences, the youngster might proceed to launch into an extensive description of his favorite car engine, oblivious to the social codes surrounding a church service.

Another common feature consists of the introduction of unrelated comments in the midst of an ongoing conversation, perhaps word associations or fragments memorized from a previous dialogue or a favorite story or film. Such interruptions can be frustrating for the unsuspecting conversational partner, and tend to increase the child's social isolation.

Additionally, children with AS struggle with prosody, an unusual rhythm, stress, pattern, or pitch. They may talk in a flat, high-pitched, sing-song, or mechanically robotic tone of voice. As a result, an AS child's intonation pattern may be incongruent with what the child wishes to communicate. Likewise, rhythm and stress on particular words may be off, giving the mistaken impression that English is a second language.

Apparent lack of empathy

Due to deficits in social communication, kids with AS may be perceived as aloof and uncaring. They may appear wooden and awkward during interactions and fail to respond with the expected facial expressions or body language when someone expresses emotion to them. However, this should not be interpreted as an inability to care for others or to experience emotion, but rather that the emotions of others in their lives may be confusing, and they may not know how to respond. Likewise, their expression of emotion may be different than it is for NT people. As an additional emotional challenge, children with AS may become overwhelmed by strong emotions, even positive ones. They may become "flooded" and shut down, not being able to figure out what to do or say.

Minimal eye contact

Lack of eye contact is one of the most overt social difficulties for many AS children. Meeting eye to eye might make the child feel acutely uncomfortable, or even terrified, and such direct contact is often deliberately avoided. Although NTs may not be aware of it, eye contact contributes a significant amount of information during a social exchange. This additional stimulation may be distracting for the child with AS, since trying to comprehend verbal information while maintaining eye contact may, in fact, break his concentration. Some adults with AS have likened making eye contact to watching one hundred televisions at once! As a result, an AS child is likely to look away or even close his eyes during conversation, often to the consternation and bewilderment of the person with whom he is speaking.

Restricted repertoire of interests

The propensity to become utterly engrossed by a special interest that dominates the person's time and conversational repertoire occurs to an exaggerated degree in a child with AS. These fascinations are engaged in with an intensity, exclusivity, and undivided focus that sets them apart from the favorite subjects or interests of NT children. Special interests are usually solitary and often quite arcane. The excessive nature of these preoccupations may be trying for parents and teachers alike. The focus of obsession can periodically change over months or years. Younger kids may focus all of their attention on collecting specific objects such as bottle openers, keys, pop cans or green pens. Often nothing can separate such a child from acquiring his desired item, and his highly developed radar system will uncannily hone in on the object in the most amazing places and at the most inconvenient times.

As a child becomes older, the special interest often transitions to a subject, or preoccupation. Regardless of whether the subject is spiders, train models, stars and planets, fire trucks, dinosaurs, bus schedules, or maps, the youngster accrues extraordinary amounts of raw data, facts, and statistics. He may develop an encyclopedic knowledge of the subject, reading every related book in the library, and exhausting all available sources of information.

Special interests like these are likely to serve multiple purposes for the child. As they often involve data, facts and orderly statistics, they are reliable and predictable. This type of information can be a safe haven from the onslaught of a confusing and changing world. Since conversation doesn't come easily, the youngster is likely to find himself unable to "make small talk." On the other hand, extensive knowledge of a familiar subject permits him to speak fluently and knowledgably for hours.

Need for structure and routine

Routine and structure play an immensely important role in giving a child with AS a semblance of control over his life. This desperate need for structure is especially intense when there have been life changes such as a new school, new house, or new family member. Repetition and routine may be perceived as anxiety-reducing, soothing, and pleasurable. Changes in routine, interruption, or sudden transitions may be intolerable. Your simple request that your youngster turn off the *The Lion King*, which he has watched thirty-four times, or put away his *Yugio* cards to come to dinner, may turn rapidly into an explosive episode. A change in classroom schedule or a transition from recess to art class may be met with fierce opposition and an accompanying meltdown. Your child may be so entrenched on a particular track that rerouting him may pose an insurmountable task, or at least one that is not worth the resulting mayhem. Consequences are likely to be ignored, regardless of their severity.

This need for sameness and routine is played out within social groups too, especially when it comes to rules and regulations. Once the rules have been set out, your child may rigidly enforce them, acting as the class or family policeman and becoming easily angered when anyone violates a rule. Such self-appointed "police" status does little to help him fit in with his peers, resulting in further marginalization.

Trouble fitting in

Kids with AS are typically viewed by their more socially aware peers as behaving oddly and awkwardly in social settings. They may appear eccentric and emotionally immature, and may have difficulty adapting to the complex and shifting social scene. Their awkward body language, limited facial expression or use of gestures, and peculiar gaze set them conspicuously outside of the social norm. Attempts to initiate social interaction are frequently unsuccessful. Forgoing a standard greeting such as "Hello, my name is..." they may introduce themselves by launching into a long-winded diatribe about the ten fastest trains in the world. As their ability to make and sustain friendships is limited, they are often left with feelings of bewilderment, loneliness, and defeat.

Literal to a fault
Lacking an understanding of tact, or the sophisticated, socially appropriate "white" lies that spare hurt feelings, these children may come across as overly blunt. For example, on observing an obese or disfigured person, a child with AS may loudly proclaim out how fat and ugly the person is, to the point of offering suggestions concerning weight reduction and beautification. A patient of ours once publicly corrected a classmate's grammatical error while her peer was in the midst of giving a public performance in the school auditorium. Although kids with AS may recognize their social *faux pas* once the error is explained to them, they often have difficulty generalizing this knowledge for use again in the future.

Interpreting the world literally and concretely rather than metaphorically or abstractly often causes AS children (and adults!) to see things as "black and white" with little opportunity for interpretation of "gray" areas. Such a limited way of perceiving the world may provide safety and comfort to a child with AS by helping to make the incomprehensible more "concrete." Overly literal interpretation of proverbs or common expressions such as the "cat got your tongue?" can provoke unexpected and socially aberrant reactions. A child may be able to tell you everything observable about a brown and white cow standing in a field, but absolutely nothing about the proverbial purple cow, who can not be seen in a literal fashion. The memory of what has been observed can in some cases be prodigious, even eidetic, with exquisite attention to detail, but with some difficulty in "seeing the forest for the trees." (Which, of course, is an expression many people with AS would find confusing!)

Bizarre behaviors
Habits such as picking, poking, flapping, flicking fingers, walking on toes, looking at objects sideways, or spinning can be pronounced in kids with AS. Though they may be involuntary and unnoticed on the part of the child engaged in such activities, the sheer repetitive quality of the bizarre behaviors often sets up further obstacles to fitting in with NT peers.

Difficulties with sports
During childhood and adolescence, group activities such as team sports are a common venue for establishing friendships. Children with AS may have little interest or ability in sports and games that are so often key to social acceptance on the playground and the neighborhood soccer field. These children may be clumsy and suffer deficits in muscular and hand-eye coordination. They often have limited fine and gross motor skills. Throwing, kicking, and catching balls may be difficult, if not impossible. When all of the other youngsters run off to play soccer or jump rope during recess, the AS child may wander around the periphery of the playground, absorbed in the intricacies of his own mind.

Precocious reading abilities
Children with AS may demonstrate a precocious ability to read which parallels their extensive vocabulary development. This is called *hyperlexia*. However, they have a

problem with comprehension and contextual under-standing. Although a five-year old with AS may be able to pick up the *Wall Street Journal* and begin reading aloud about a recent hike in interest rates, his comprehension of the meaning of the article will lag far behind. With hyperlexia, there is a discrepancy between one's ability to read a word and the interrelated skills involved in com-prehending the meaning of a word within its context.[4]

Physical hypersensitivity
Oversensitivity to a myriad of stimuli, including touch, texture, pressure, light, odors and tastes, is common in children with AS. Sirens, school bells, crowd noise, yelling and screaming, or even the buzz from fluorescent lights, can range from annoying to painful, causing extreme reactions that may leave those around them wondering: what just happened? Bright or blinking lights, scratchy tags on shirts, tight clothing, or seams in socks—easily ignored by all but the most sensitive NT kids—may be literally unbearable. Conversely, some people with AS have *decreased* sensitivity to stimuli, and are unruffled by or seem not to notice sensations that most NTs would consider over the top. A child with AS may have both over- and under-sensitivities. For example, she may be unable to wear socks or tight clothing, while at the same time blissfully unaware of an offensive odor or a striking change in temperature.

Many of these sensory issues cause AS kids to be described as selective or picky about food, drink, clothing, environment, objects, and people. This sel-ectivity can mightily test parents, teachers, and caregivers, who—try as they may—can't seem to please their "picky" kids.

There are youngsters who will only eat foods from a specific category like white foods, soft foods, crunchy foods, or dry foods. Others may refuse to eat mixed foods, slimy foods, or foods "contaminated" by utensils or by barely touching some other "gross" food that they consider inedible. Then there are those who will drink only milk, or pop, or a certain juice. Just imagine preparing meals for such a child each day. While all parents may occasionally run into such battles, the rigidity of AS children is legendary. Many parents simply give up and let their child survive on what he *will* eat, perhaps sneaking nutritional supplements into those few "acceptable" foods.

Fear of failure and low self-esteem

Although negative feedback is unpleasant for most of us, it may be especially painful for a child who finds himself the resident of an incomprehensible world in which he doesn't know how to play by the mostly unspoken rules. The ability to learn new things, generalize learning, adapt to new and shifting situations, and learn from one's mistakes is often crucial for success in social and school situations. Because of their rigidity, youngsters with AS may repeatedly fail. This inability to adapt and be flexible may trigger ongoing criticism.

An Alternative Path Helps the Stranger Return Home

Hopefully, the catalogue of characteristics above has piqued your interest in AS, or reminded you of experiences you've had as a teacher, parent, or caregiver of such a child. Perhaps you fit the AS profile yourself. As we explore the multi-faceted world of children and adults with AS throughout this book, we hope to show you how, with the help of homeopathic medicine, being a "stranger in a strange land" can be transformed into the familiar feeling of arriving home. Conventional doctors often use psychiatric medication to assist in this process. Sometimes medication is presented as the only option. Though medications have their place and can be helpful at times with some target symptoms, we offer a viable alternative to prescription drugs. In the next chapter, we provide an overview of the psychiatric drugs used to treat ASD, and, where available, the research supporting the use of these various medications. We will then introduce you to homeopathy, which we have found to be the most effective alternative to conventional drugs.

2

Better Living through Chemistry?

The Pros and Cons of Medication

One of the most difficult decisions parents will make is whether or not to use psychotropic (psychiatric) medication to treat an ASD child. For some children, medications are the missing link, and can make an undeniable difference. For others, the side effects are unbearable, or the drugs simply don't work. The decision to medicate your child depends on a number of factors. Unfortunately, there isn't one right answer that fits all children.

Billy's Story*

Billy, an intelligent and curious third grader, had trouble deciphering interactions with his peers. They might as well be speaking a different language, one that he had not had the opportunity to learn. When he attempted to play with the other students, they would often just walk away, making disparaging remarks that baffled Billy. When they laughed and joked among themselves, Billy wondered if they were laughing at him because the jokes didn't seem very logical or funny. Billy desperately

---

* While all of the cases in Part II of this book are drawn directly from our practice, we have taken the liberty in this section to include composite, fictional cases, such as Billy's, for educational purposes.

wanted to be part of the group, but despite multiple ill-fated attempts, he just couldn't figure out how to fit in. Although the adults at school were kind and would talk to him, he could still claim no friends among his peers. As the school year progressed, Billy became increasingly more perplexed about what he was doing wrong. As Billy's desperation increased, his confusion deepened, and he started to become angry. When the other students ignored or rejected his overtures, he sometimes grabbed them and occasionally threw them to the ground.

As a result, Billy began spending more time in the principal's office. Additionally, the parents of Billy's classmates were calling the school to complain about his rough-housing. It was only a matter of time before his mom received a call from the school psychologist requesting a meeting. With a sinking feeling, Billy's parents entered the conference room to be greeted by the psychologist, the principal, and Billy's homeroom teacher. They could tell this was serious, and as they sat down, they waited for the other shoe to drop.

Billy's father questioned the psychologist and the principal: *"Is Billy's rough-housing really over the top? Or is this school district particularly strict? Don't all third grade boys play rough? I was like that when I was a kid too. Let boys be boys!"* But Billy's mom wasn't so sure. Maybe there is something to this, she thought. *"I've been receiving angry calls from other moms who tell me that their sons have been hurt by Billy,"* she told the group.

The school psychologist expressed the feeling that Billy's aggression had crossed the line, and that he had hurt some of his classmates. *"I don't think that Billy is an aggressive child by nature,"* she offered, *"but his aggression seems to be escalating."* Billy's mom responded, *"We are just as baffled by Billy's behavior. We have a peaceful home, and Billy has never acted like this before. In fact, at home, he is a very sweet, mild, and extremely helpful child.*"

Despite Billy's parents assertions, the school psychologist continued to push her agenda and inquired, "*Has Billy ever been to a child psychiatrist? Have you considered putting him on medication? We are concerned that Billy may not be able to remain in the mainstream classroom if his behaviors continue,*" she added, as she offered a referral to a local child psychiatrist.

Billy's parents sulked out of the room, bewildered and feeling like they had been set up. They didn't know whether to feel anger toward the school or at Billy for letting himself, and them, down. Or, even whether to blame themselves for some imagined deficiency in their parenting skills. Though uneasy with the psychologist's recommendation, they felt under pressure to make an appointment with the psychiatrist and to medicate Billy. They felt as if the school had forced them into a medical paradigm with which they felt highly uncomfortable. Unfortunately, this scenario is all too frequent.

Clearly, in Billy's case, what lay beneath his angry behavior was his inability to form relationships with or to comprehend his peers. The desperation of not being part of the group made Billy angry and sometimes aggressive. Although the root of the problem is social impairment, conventional psychiatric treatment targets only the *effect*, aggression.

Currently, there is no conventional cure for ASD. Furthermore, it is important to realize that no psychotropic medications specifically address the core symptoms of ASD. While medications may sometimes address isolated symptoms and control unwanted behaviors such as attention problems, aggression, ritualistic or stereotyped behaviors, and anxiety, they fail to treat the core symptoms of ASD.

Overmedication of Children:
A Growing Concern

A study conducted by Dr. Julie Zito at the University of Maryland, published in 2003, emphasized the alarming increase in the number of American children who are being treated by psychiatric drugs.[5] Zito reported that from 1987 to 1996, the number of medicated children not only tripled, but showed no sign of slowing down.[6]

In her study, Zito expressed concern that cost-saving techniques by insurance companies, marketing by the pharmaceutical industry, and increased demands on parents and doctors may be behind the steep rise in the use of medication with children. Who benefits from this trend? The children? Or is it the insurance companies and the pharmaceutical industry? The study goes on to state that, other than "zonking" unmanageable kids, it is questionable that management by drug control yields lasting changes in behavior.[7] Furthermore, though drugs may dampen objectionable behavior, they do not address the underlying problem if a child does not know how to properly handle social interactions. Zito's concerns speak directly to the medicating of ASD children.

The FDA and Off-Label Prescribing

Surprisingly, nearly all of the psychotropic medications prescribed for children with ASD lack official approval by the Food and Drug Administration (FDA) for the treatment of it. Just because a drug is on the market and being prescribed by doctors does not necessarily mean that it has been proven safe and effective for the treated condition. In fact, a majority of the psychiatric drugs used to treat ASD have not undergone rigorous testing for safety or effectiveness, and very few of them have been tested at all in children. Fortunately, it's to our children's benefit that researchers are now beginning to carefully examine the appropriateness of medication for each individual child.[8]

Many drugs are used to treat conditions other than what they were originally designed to treat. For example, Tenex (Guanfacine HCL), a drug originally developed to treat high blood pressure, is also used to treat tic disorders in children. Using drugs in this manner is referred to as off-label prescribing. Though not illegal, it is a risky and very controversial practice. Off-label prescribing is very common with children, especially for treating those with ASD.

Medications Do Have a Place

Although psychiatric medications don't offer a cure for ASD, and may be risky for some children, when properly indicated and used under close supervision, they can be helpful in addressing specific behavioral problems such as depression, obsessive-compulsive disorder or anxiety. Some of the more commonly prescribed categories of drugs follow:

Stimulants (Adderal, Concerta, Cyclert, Dexedrine, Ritalin)

Stimulant medications are the most commonly prescribed class of drugs for children as a whole. Although up to 75% of children with ASD have been on them at some point, they have not been extensively studied in individuals with autism.[9] Most commonly, this class of drugs is prescribed for symptoms related to Attention Deficit Hyperactivity Disorder (ADHD) and Attention Deficit Disorder (ADD).

Antidepressants (Celexa, Luvox, Paxil, Prozac, Zoloft)
Selective serotonin reuptake inhibitors (SSRIs) are the most commonly prescribed drugs for people with pervasive developmental disorders. Although they are well known for the treatment of depression in adults, they have not consistently been proven safe or effective for treating depression in children. Recently, a panel of experts recommended to the FDA that ten antidepressant drugs be given a "black box" warning, the government's strongest safety alert, on their prescribing labels. The expert panel supported their recommendation with multiple studies indicating that children and teenagers who take antidepressants are *twice* as likely as those given placebos to become suicidal.[10] Additionally, the panel cited that "most of the drugs failed in studies to ameliorate the symptoms of depression in teenagers and children."[11]

In the treatment of ASD, SSRIs are used to address repetitive behaviors, anxiety, insomnia, and compulsions. For some children, they may be helpful in addressing these target symptoms. For others, the potential for suicidal behavior and lack of effectiveness outweigh the benefits. Unfortunately, physicians currently have no method for distinguishing between these two groups.

Mood stabilizers (Depakote, Dilantin, Eskalith, Lithobid, Neurontin, Tegretol)
This class of medications is the first-line treatment for adults with bipolar disorder. Although a few studies have been conducted on adolescents without ASD concerning the use of lithium (Eskalith, Lithobid, Lithonate), absolutely no double-blind studies have been conducted to date on its effectiveness or safety for children with ASD. And even less information is available concerning other mood stabilizers. In general, lithium has not been

shown to have beneficial effects for treating the core symptoms of autism.[12]

With lithium, there is a fine line between the therapeutic level and a toxic level. Because lithium toxicity is a serious and potentially fatal condition, there is a need for routine blood work. Not surprisingly, children with the common hypersensitivities of ASD often have a strong aversion to having their blood drawn, thus making toxicity evaluation difficult.

Antihypertensives (Tenex, Catapres)

Originally developed to treat high blood pressure, antihypertensive drugs are also used off-label with ASD children to treat aggression, tics, impulsivity, agitation, and sleep problems. Because these medications have systemic effects on cardiovascular function, they must be closely monitored. To date, none of these medications has been rigorously studied for use with children on the autism continuum.

Antipsychotics (Risperdal, Zyprexa, Geodon, Abilify)

Originally designed to treat thought disorders such as psychosis and schizophrenia, antipsychotics (also known as neuroleptics) are increasingly being used off-label to control difficult behaviors in children with ASD. Few studies have carefully evaluated the efficacy and safety of antipsychotic agents for children and adolescents.

Recently, a serious concern surrounding the use of antipsychotic drugs has arisen: researchers have established the side effect of significant weight gain and a greater risk for diabetes. In a recent study on treating autism with Risperdal, children on the drug gained weight at alarming rates—on average, six pounds over eight weeks. Even after the six-month point in the study, the weight gain continued, unabated.[13] We have observed this weight gain ourselves in some of our patients who have been prescribed antipsychotics by other health professionals. Obesity only compounds the obvious difficulties met by youngsters with ASD in regards to making friends and being accepted by their classmates.

To Drug or Not to Drug

All parents want to see their kids healthy and happy, and many are reluctant to place their ASD child on psychiatric medications. Parents are often under enormous pressure from the educational or medical communities to medicate their children. Intimidated by so much pressure, they may feel they have no other options, that prescription drugs are the only answer. This is not true. You and your child *do* have a choice.

We've helped many children and adults avoid or taper off psychiatric medications through the use of homeopathy. We know that these remedies are safe and effective—and much gentler than the alternative. There isn't any one easy solution for ASD, but the answer to your child's (or your own) problems may be found in the pages of this book.

Homeopathy
Medicine for All of You

Suppose, for a moment, that you were to pick up a newspaper and the headlines were to read: *Revolutionary New Medicine Holds Promise for Humanity.* As you read the article, you discover that this "revolutionary" medicine is:

- A well-proven alternative successfully used for over 200 years
- Natural and largely free of side effects
- Extraordinarily safe
- Effective in treating physical, mental, emotional, and behavioral problems
- Highly individualized treatment based on more than just the diagnosis
- Able to show evidence of improvement in many cases of ASD
- Practiced by professionals who take the time to listen and understand you and your child
- More affordable than conventional medications
- Covered by some insurance providers
- Individualized to the specific needs of each child
- Working in harmony with the body's natural healing process
- Able to prevent disease
- Supported by numerous double-blind studies

- Practiced throughout the world
- Over 2,000 medicines available
- Compatible with conventional medications
- Used and endorsed by a number of politicians, celebrities, and professional athletes
- Available to you and your family right now!

Wouldn't You Want to Go Right Out and Try It?

Wouldn't you be at least mildly curious? Or maybe even wildly curious? What if you or a loved one were diagnosed with ASD, or some other serious health concern, and did not feel comfortable taking conventional medications? Wouldn't you want to know more about such a medicine? If so, read on!

❦ *Homeopathy is a well-proven alternative successfully used for 200 years*
Although homeopathy was developed 200 years ago by German physician and scholar Samuel Hahnemann, the underlying principles date back to the time of the Greek physician Hippocrates (450 B.C.). Hahnemann, also a chemist and medical translator, sought a method of healing that was safe, natural, effective, and much gentler than the rather crude medical methods in use in the early 19th century. Medicine in those days involved purging, bloodletting, and the use of leeches and strong, poisonous chemicals like mercury and arsenic. Hahnemann felt that the doctors of his time often did more harm than good, and he could no longer bear to practice that way. Through extensive research, some of it performed on himself, he determined a basic principle of healing, which he called the *Law of Similars*, or more simply, "like cures like." The

Law of Similars says that whatever symptoms a substance from nature will produce when given to a healthy person, it can heal in a person who is ill.

Natural substances are specially prepared as homeopathic medicines through a process of successive dilutions, and are given in small doses. For example, the homeopathic medicine *Apis* (most homeopathic medicines have Latin names) is derived from the honeybee. When a person suffers a bee sting, *Apis* will significantly reduce the pain, inflammation and swelling. The reason for this is that these are the very symptoms that a bee sting causes in a healthy person. *Apis* can also be effective in treating this same constellation of symptoms if they are associated with conjunctivitis, allergic reactions, arthritis, or bladder infections.

❧ Homeopathic medicines are natural and largely free of side effects

All but a few homeopathic medicines are derived from natural substances, rather than being synthetically produced like most conventional drugs. In preparing the medicine, this natural substance is diluted again and again—so often, in fact, that there may only be a few molecules of the original substance remaining in the homeopathic medicine. Though the principle by which homeopathic medicines are prescribed is well understood and clinically tested, the precise mechanism of action is still under investigation.

Homeopathic medicines do not usually produce side effects in the conventional sense of the word. However, an aggravation, or temporary worsening of existing symptoms may occur. An aggravation typically begins within a few days to a week of taking the medicine and rarely lasts more than a few weeks. Infrequently, in extremely sensitive people, symptoms characteristic of the medicine may transiently appear. As soon as the medicine is discontinued, the symptoms will disappear.

❧ *Homeopathic medicines are extraordinarily safe*
When properly prescribed, homeopathic medicines have a gentle yet powerful action. When an incorrect medicine is administered, it generally has no effect at all. Homeopathic medicines have been used safely by infants, pregnant women, and the elderly for over two centuries. Homeopathy is an excellent choice of medicine for people who are highly sensitive to foods, medications, vaccines, or the environment.

❧ *Homeopathy is effective in treating physical,*
mental, emotional, and behavioral problems
Homeopathy is as effective in treating most mental and emotional conditions as it is in treating physical problems. We have seen positive results for chronic conditions such as allergies, eczema, asthma, upper respiratory infections, and digestive problems, as well as acute illnesses like colds, flu, sore throats, and ear infections. We have found homeopathy to be highly effective for developmental, behavioral, and psychiatric conditions such as AS, ADHD, depression, anxiety, OCD, panic attacks, and mood swings, as well as other behavioral and learning problems.

❧ *Homeopathy offers highly individualized treatment*
based on more than just the diagnosis
Although diagnostic labels are recognized by homeopaths as communicating the common symptoms of a particular illness, they serve only as a beginning point for a homeopathic prescription. Homeopaths look for individualizing symptoms specific to the person experiencing the illness. We are far more interested in how your child, diagnosed

with ASD is different from every other child with the same diagnosis.

Let's use the analogy of a jigsaw puzzle. Suppose that the puzzles of two children both resemble animals. A homeopath will narrow the focus to which *type* of animal. If it is clear that both pictures depict dinosaurs, we then need to identify which particular kind of dinosaur. Once all the pieces are assembled, one puzzle might ultimately represent a velociraptor and the other a T-rex. Similar dinosaurs, but not quite the same! This is the work of the homeopath—to decide which single homeopathic medicine best matches that person's unique "picture" of symptoms and behaviors.

❦ *Homeopathy is able to show evidence of improvement in many cases of ASD*

Positive personal experience, or at least hearing about other people's direct experience, is what has convinced most people of homeopathy's effectiveness. In her book *Impossible Cure*, former-NASA scientist-turned-homeopath Amy Lansky, Ph.D., recounts the experience of her autistic child being cured by homeopathy. She had read Dr. Reichenberg-Ullman's article on childhood behavior problems in *Mothering* magazine and found a homeopath near her home in California to prescribe for her son.

> *Our younger son, Max was inexplicably afflicted with autism. This tragic and supposedly incurable disorder dramatically limits a child's ability to communicate and connect with others. And for some reason, it is mysteriously striking more and more children every year. Given the limited options for treatment, we were coping as best we could.*
>
> *By January of 1999, only four years later, everything had changed. I was now the mother of two*

sons progressing nicely through grade school. Max was no longer autistic—he was bright, talkative and sociable. His autism had been cured with a controversial medicine of the past—homeopathy.[14]

❦ Homeopathy is practiced by professionals who take the time to listen and understand you and your child

We schedule two hours for an initial appointment for a child. Contrast this with the typically briefer initial interview with a pediatrician or psychiatrist, and you can easily see how a homeopath may come to develop more in-depth knowledge of your child. At first, you might wonder whether your child would even be willing to talk to someone like us. And, for some kids, especially more severely autistic children, you may be right. There are many cases where the child is either unable or unwilling to communicate verbally. But you would be surprised how freely most children will talk with us, especially once they understand that there are no right or wrong answers in a homeopathic interview.

A homeopath is genuinely interested in what makes your child tick, and delights in engaging in conversation about her favorite topic, whether it is oscillating fans, trains or planes, or Bionicles. Everything that strongly captures her attention also captures ours. Parents routinely tell us that their children talk more freely to us than to any doctor they have seen, and we find that they feel safe and comfortable enough to reveal information unknown even to their parents.

❦ Homeopathic medicines are more affordable than conventional medications

Although the initial visit with a homeopath may cost as much as consulting with another type of specialist, the cost of the medicine is far lower. A year's supply of homeopathic medicine for your child is likely to be less expensive than a one-month prescription of even a single psychiatric medication. Homeopathic visits are rarely more frequent than six to eight weeks apart, even in the beginning of treatment. As your child gets better, the visits become even more infrequent, only scheduled two to four times a year.

❦ *Homeopathy is covered by some insurance providers*
A growing number of third-party carriers are now reimbursing for homeopathic care. Whether or not your homeopathic practitioner is covered will depend largely on the medical licensure requirements and policy provisions of your particular insurance carrier. Homeopathic treatment is generally billed as an office visit rather than called a homeopathic interview. The diagnostic code assigned may also determine the whether the care provided is eligible for reimbursement. Since some insurance carriers specifically exclude care for a child diagnosed with autism, you should call your insurance company before your child's first homeopathic appointment to ask specific questions about your particular insurance policy's requirements for homeopathic care.

Telephone consultations with a homeopath are less likely to be covered than in-person consultations. Even if homeopathy is not reimbursable under your policy, it may count towards your deductible. We believe that those without insurance coverage will still find that treatment by a qualified and experienced homeopath is well worth the out-of-pocket expense.

❦ *Homeopathic treatment is individualized to the specific needs of each child*
Because homeopathic medicines are so highly individualized, ten different children with AS are likely to be prescribed ten entirely different homeopathic medicines. A

key advantage of homeopathy is that the medicine is much more specific and tailored to the exact symptoms of your child than even the most accurately prescribed pharmaceutical drugs. While psychiatric medications are likely to treat only your child's narrowly defined target symptoms rather than the underlying AS, homeopathy treats the whole child, whatever her diagnosis. When the child is addressed as a whole, both the common and the unique symptoms will likely diminish, sometimes dramatically.

❦ Homeopathy works in harmony with the body's natural healing process

Much of the thrust of traditional Western medicine is helping the body "fight" disease. Medications such as antibiotics, anti-inflammatories, antidepressants, anxiolytics, antipsychotics, or immunosuppressants are categorized as working against microorganisms or disease processes. The assumption is that the body is out of control, and measures must be taken to counteract the physiological processes causing symptoms such as infection, inflammation, depression, anxiety, or psychosis.

In contrast, homeopathy works *with* the body's natural healing tendencies rather than *opposing* them, bringing the body back into balance as a whole rather than trying to suppress individual "problem" symptoms. Healing occurs naturally once the body and mind are restored to equilibrium.

❦ Homeopathy is able to prevent disease

Children who are treated successfully with homeopathy are less vulnerable to infectious diseases, allergies, and acute childhood illnesses. Parents of our patients often tell us that the kids we've treated remain well, even while the rest of the family or playmates come down

with one illness after another. Not only are acute illnesses less prevalent among homeopathic patients, but we
have found our patients to experience fewer chronic illnesses as well.

❦ Homeopathy is supported by numerous double-blind studies

Some medical doctors and those grounded in evidence-
based medicine criticize homeopathy for lacking double-
blind studies or attribute its healing effect to placebo.
These critiques are simply false and most often reveal an
unscientific bias. While research funds and access to conventional academic research settings for homeopathy are
limited, over one hundred high-quality, randomized,
placebo-controlled studies do exist, many showing positive outcomes for homeopathic treatment.

In a 1994 issue of *Pediatrics*, Jennifer Jacobs, MD,
published a placebo-controlled study of the homeopathic
treatment of diarrhea in Nicaragua.[15] Homeopathic treatment made a statistically significant difference in com-
parison with the placebo group. The group treated with
homeopathy clearly showed a shortened duration of the
disease's course, on average by about one day.

More recently, Jacobs et al. published another
randomized placebo-controlled study of the homeopathic
treatment of acute otitis media (ear infection) in children.[16] Overall, there were nearly 20% more treatment
failures in the placebo group than in the homeopathic
group. Although parents were allowed to give pain relievers to their children, children in the placebo group needed the pain relievers twice as frequently as those in the
homeopathic group.

Finally, two significant meta-analyses have been
published in prestigious British medical journals. Most
recently, Dr. Klaus Linde demonstrated that homeopathy,

on average, was nearly 250% more effective than place-bo.[17] Linde's study included eighty-nine randomized, placebo-controlled studies while excluding all single-case studies. Another meta-analysis published in 1991 scientifically demonstrated that the effects of homeopathic medicine far exceed those of placebo effect.[18]

Though we have presented only a small sample of the high-quality, scientifically rigorous studies that have been conducted on homeopathy, we encourage you to explore and keep abreast of this growing field of research.

❦ Homeopathy is practiced throughout the world
In Europe, South America and India, homeopathy enjoys far greater acceptance than it does in the United States. Every French pharmacy carries homeopathic medicine, and homeopathy is practiced throughout the European Union. According to the Boiron Group, one of the world's leading manufacturers of homeopathics, sales of homeopathic medicine amount to more than a billion euros per year worldwide, with France alone accounting for 230 million euros in sales per year.

Homeopathy is practiced in 80 countries throughout the world, including most nations in Europe and the Americas, Israel, India, Pakistan, Sri Lanka, Australia, New Zealand, and South Africa. Homeopathy is a regular part of the national health systems of Britain, France, Germany, Norway, Greece, India, Israel, and Austria. In India alone there are 120 homeopathic medical schools and over 100,000 practitioners who routinely treat serious diseases such as tuberculosis, typhoid, malaria, leprosy, hepatitis, and HIV homeopathically.

❦ Homeopathy has over 2,000 available medicines
Homeopathic medicines come from every corner of the natural world, including the mineral, plant, and animal

kingdoms. Minerals such as table salt, gold, and diamond are used, as well as plants such as jasmine, cedar, and oregano. Animal sources such as the tarantula spider, dolphin's milk, and Gila monster also provide the raw materials for medicines. There is an active and dynamic process worldwide of introducing new, carefully tested substances to the homeopathic repertoire. Homeopathic pharmacies take great care to extract the samples used to make the medicines with as little harm possible.

❦ *Homeopathic medicines are compatible with conventional medications*
Homeopathic medicines will not interfere with conventional medications your child may be taking, but your doctor may not be aware of this. Many of our patients are already taking pharmaceutical drugs when they begin homeopathic treatment, particularly psychiatric medications. In many cases, as your child's symptoms improve through homeopathic care, it may be possible, under the guidance of the prescribing physician, to slowly decrease the dosage of drugs or to discontinue them entirely.

❦ *Homeopathy is used and endorsed by a number of politicians, celebrities, and professional athletes*
Many well-known and respected people in the political, entertainment, and business worlds are proponents of homeopathic medicine. Mahatma Gandhi, Yehudi Menuhin, Bill Clinton, the British Royal Family, Boris Becker, David Beckham, Martina Navratilova, Pat Riley, Lindsay Wagner, Catherine Zeta-Jones, Pamela Anderson, Jane Fonda, Martin Sheen, Whoopi Goldberg, Cher, Rosie O'Donnell, Nick Nolte, Ashley and Naomi Judd, Lisa Marie-Presley, Tina Turner, and Paul McCartney have all come out publicly in support of homeopathy. Many others choose to remain anonymous, but may still contribute

to the growth of the field in other ways.

❦ *Homeopathy is available to you and your family right now*

Homeopathic medicine is practiced by a wide variety of practitioners, including:

- naturopathic physicians (ND)
- certified, professional homeopaths (RS Hom., NA)
- medical doctors (MD)
- osteopaths, (DO)
- chiropractors (DC)
- nurses (RN) and family nurse practitioners (FNP)
- physician's assistants (PA)
- acupuncturists (LAc)
- dentists (DDS)
- veterinarians (DVM)

As of this writing, the United States has fewer than a thousand homeopathic practitioners, a fraction of the number of medical doctors and other health care professionals. But the number is growing steadily. As there are still many states and localities in the U.S. where there are no qualified and experienced homeopathic practitioners, a significant portion of our own practice is conducted by telephone consultation.

4

Homeopathy for ASD
Exceptional Medicine for Exceptional Kids

Homeopathy may be unique and unconventional medicine, but it can produce exceptional changes in children with ASD. Not only can homeopathy address the social, learning, and behavioral problems typical of ASD, but it also can help many acute and chronic health problems.

Since homeopathy treats the whole person, it takes into account all of the factors that make up your child's unique blend of symptoms and behaviors, likes and dislikes. Because homeopaths individualize treatment, there is not one homeopathic medicine used for all cases of ASD. Instead, a homeopath's job is to match the child to one of over 2,000 medicines. In this chapter we will cover how homeopathy is a good match for your ASD child, how the correct medicine is found, and what to expect from a course of homeopathic treatment.

Why ASD Children are Excellent Candidates for Homeopathic Care

❧ *The more unusual the child, the easier it is to help him with homeopathy*
The more features that differentiate one child from all others, the easier it is to identify the one "matching" medicine. It is far more difficult to find the correct

medicine for a NT child with run-of-the-mill allergies than it is for a child with ASD, most of whom are quite unusual. Whenever we hear a feature or symptom that we have never before heard, it intrigues us. Unusual symptoms or behaviors narrow down the possibilities in choosing the correct medicine from over 2,000 medicines.

❧ **Homeopathy is gentle medicine for super-sensitive kids**
Many ASD children are highly sensitive to prescription drugs, foods, and other substances. Since the ingredients in homeopathic medicines are so highly diluted, allergic reactions, sensitivities, or even side effects are rare. Homeopathy is one of the gentlest forms of medicine known. A few children do react adversely in some way to homeopathic medicines, but virtually all such reactions can be minimized or eliminated by an alternative form of dosing.

❧ **Homeopathic medicines pass the taste test**
ASD kids are often extraordinarily picky about what they will eat. The smallest amount of nutritional supplements, whether given in capsules, liquids or hidden in foods, is often easily detected and adamantly refused. In contrast, many children enjoy taking their homeopathic medicine and ask for more!

❧ **A homeopath does not need to physically examine a child to prescribe a homeopathic medicine**
Hypersensitive kids often find being touched, especially by strangers, extremely uncomfortable. We rely on the child's pediatrician to perform physical examinations, draw blood, and give shots as needed. This allows us to maintain a therapeutic relationship as the child's ally and confidante rather than someone who inflicts pain or causes discomfort.

❦ *The homeopathic interview is a perfect opportunity to talk about grand passions*

Homeopaths love to engage kids in a lively discussion of their favorite subjects or activities. Even more than the background information parents may give, hearing the child talk about what fascinates him, observing his gestures and body language, and listening for impassioned tones of voice can lead a homeopath directly to the right medicine. Every word the child utters is of significance to us, particularly words or language that are unique. Whereas parents, teachers, and caregivers may roll their eyes if they hear even once more about the cube root of 4096, our eyes light up, and we record the words of the child feverishly, trying not to miss a single word.

❦ *Homeopathic interviews can be fun!*

Our office is filled with toys, games, stuffed animals, and two sweet golden retrievers who win over many a wary child. When kids are able to relax and play a little before and during the interview, it often puts them in a good mood, and soon they begin to look forward to seeing us. The child has an opportunity, if willing, to speak with us alone. We recognize and appreciate each child as a valuable, interesting individual. In person or by phone, we give youngsters a chance to say what they want, discuss their dreams and fears, share what interests them such as movies, books or video games, and to describe their most cherished ideas, thoughts or fantasies. We show a genuine interest in them, and they know it. Our main objective is not to try to find a diagnostic cubbyhole in which to place them or to perform psychological testing, but rather, simply try to get to know them for who they are. (Homeopaths do not conduct formal psychological or IQ testing for diagnosing ASD, so if you want those tests done, please consult a pediatric or school psychologist or another appropriate professional.)

❦ *Highly motivated parents are a homeopath's dream*
Parents of children with ASD are highly motivated to find
help for their kids, willing to go to any extent to help their
children, including searching for any treatment that can
turn around their youngsters' symptoms and disabilities.
They are willing to travel long distances to get the best
possible treatment, sometimes even flying across country
to see us. All told, parents of children on the autism spectrum tend to be committed to their child's treatment and
well being for the long haul.

Typically, one parent hears about homeopathy first
and introduces it to the other. It is not uncommon for the
mother, for example, to feel strongly, after reading one of
our books, that homeopathy is the route for her child.
The father may agree to the plan quite readily, or may be
more reluctant. It is not necessary for both parents to
have the same conviction that homeopathy will work for
their child, but it is essential that everyone who is inti-
mately involved with the child is willing to provide as
much information as possible to the homeopath. When
both parents are on board for the treatment journey, the
odds of success are significantly increased.

❦ *Homeopathic visits are infrequent*
Compared to most of the other therapies you will engage
in, homeopathic visits are infrequent (typically 6 to 8
weeks apart or more) and will not tax your already full
schedule. We realize that parents of ASD kids are often
stretched to the max, driving their children from a doctor's appointment to a speech therapy session to a social-
skills group. Add to this their siblings' activities, highly
complicated meal preparation for picky eaters or children
on special diets, and you have a recipe for stress.

❦ *Homeopathic interviews can be conducted by phone*
Conducting homeopathic interviews by phone can be a
blessing for parents and children with ASD. We recognize that many parents have difficulty traveling with
their ASD children. Transitions are difficult for many of
these children, making arriving on time for a scheduled
appointment a real challenge. Additionally, some children
prefer phone consultations because they fear face-to- face
interactions with strangers.

The Homeopathic Interview

It's helpful to know what to expect before taking your
child to his initial homeopathic appointment. Before the
visit, you will be asked to fill out a medical history form,
which will help your practitioner gain an overview of
issues regarding your child that may not come up spontaneously during the interview. Then, be prepared to
spend two hours with your homeopathic practitioner.
Exact times may vary, but this is a typical average. Be
sure to arrive a bit early to take care of paperwork with
the office staff.

The first visit is a unique and vital opportunity for
your homeopath to get to know you and your child. You
are investing precious time, money, and trust in your
child's treatment. Make the most of it.

We urge you to bring another family member or
caregiver so you can devote your full, undivided attention
to the appointment. This is true for phone consultations
as well as in-person appointments. Usually, we spend the
first hour with the parent(s) alone. The child is either in
the waiting room or, in the case of phone consultations,
in a separate area of the house, so it is helpful to have
another adult looking after him. It is essential that you, as

parents, have the ability to speak freely about your child without being overheard.

During the actual interview, the homeopath will be most interested in the following points:

• physical, mental, and emotional symptoms
• behavior
• how your child gets along in the family, at school, and in other settings
• communication and speech
• words, phrases, expressions, or images that your child uses often
• special interests and favorite activities
• any particular sensitivities
• strong food and drink preferences or aversions
• relevant family history
• significant information regarding pregnancy and birth
• precipitating events or suspected causative factors related to your child's condition
• reports from teachers or school personnel, such as speech and language pathologists, psychologists, psychiatrists, paraprofessionals, and other caregivers
• fears
• dreams
• anything that you can think of that is unique or unusual about your child.

During the interview, your homeopath will mainly be listening and gathering information. Practitioners use a variety of styles when conducting the initial interview. Some homeopaths primarily listen, while others more actively question you and your child. Still others engage in a process of free association based on the precise words of the patient. All of these approaches help the homeopath assemble the pieces of the jigsaw puzzle that make up your child.

After gathering initial information from the parent(s), your homeopath will attempt to interview your child, depending on the child's ability to communicate. A great deal of useful information may be gleaned from talking with more verbal children, but observation of nonverbal gestures and behavior are equally important in finding the correct medicine for your child. Whenever possible, we encourage parents to bring their child for the initial appointment and follow up visits. If that's not possible, we ask them to provide photographs or even video clips of characteristic behaviors, to help us get a better view of the "whole picture." Even though observation is important, we have found equal success, in most cases, in interviews based upon telephone consultation with an observant parent.

Once both the parents and the child (when possible) have been interviewed, it is time for the homeopath to analyze the case and prescribe. If the pattern of symptoms in the case obviously indicates a particular homeopathic medicine, your homeopath will administer it right there in the office (or send it by mail if the child isn't present). If more study is needed to determine the correct medicine, your homeopath has homework to do. He may call you with additional questions, schedule additional time, or ask you to submit more information that would be helpful in choosing the right medicine.

The homeopathic medicine will be in a powdered, pellet, or liquid form, administered in either a single or sometimes in a daily dose. Read any instructions or recommendations carefully; they will be very different from those given with pharmaceutical drugs.

What Happens Next?

During the first week or so after your child takes the homeopathic medicine, you may notice some changes. You may simply find that his symptoms steadily improve. This immediate improvement may mean that the correct remedy was found, and the child is beginning to heal.

Sometimes within the first days or first week, existing symptoms may temporarily worsen. This is called "aggravation" and generally only occurs when the correct medicine has been given. Aggravation is a positive sign! This temporary worsening will promptly be followed by an improvement of symptoms, sometimes a dramatic change for the better.

If the medicine given is not the correct one for that patient, there is typically no response at all. If there is only a brief positive response, the medicine may either be on the mark but simply not strong enough, another dose may be needed, or a different medicine may be indicated.

Another possible response, which occurs only when the correct medicine has been given, is a fleeting return of symptoms from the past, usually lasting three to four days. This is also a very good sign. By the five- to six-week point, it should be clear to both you and your homeopath whether the medicine has acted and your child is improving.

Follow-up Visits

You will be instructed to make a follow-up appointment for about six weeks after your child begins treatment. In the weeks leading up to that visit, observe and record any changes that you or others notice. Jot down comments each day in a small notebook. Over time, it's easy to forget changes in sleep disturbances, good (or bad) days at school, sensitivity to textures and smells, etc. You are your homeopath's eyes and ears, and your notes will help him help your child. At the first follow-up visit, all of the concerns raised in the first interview will be assessed to determine what has changed, and how significantly. If no changes are evident, and the action of the medicine was not interrupted prematurely, then the homeopath will gather more information, ask more questions, and probably prescribe a different medicine. Do not be concerned if the correct medicine is not found during the first visit. Homeopaths choose from over 2,000 medicines, some of them generally similar but subtly different. It can take time to understand a child in depth, so finding the perfect match sometimes takes more than one try. Some parents become impatient when there is no change after two to three weeks, wanting to try a different medicine right away, but your homeopath must wait long enough to make sure the medicine has been given sufficient time to act. If your child responded very well initially, then the medicine seemed to stop acting, a repetition of the original dose or a stronger dose may be required.

Sometimes additional interview time may be needed to help your homeopath understand your child more completely. In some cases, it may take several tries over three to six months to find the correct homeopathic medicine. The odds are that if you continue treatment for a year, your homeopath will very likely find a medicine that gives you results, even if some trial and error is needed.

The more your homeopath knows about your child, the better the chances are of finding the correct medicine. Some of the medicines for children with ASD are relatively rare and may not be obvious to your homeopath in the beginning of treatment. If you can keep observing your child at every opportunity, and report those observations accurately, you may say something that provides your homeopath with just the clue that is needed to find the right prescription.

Once the correct medicine has been found, appointments will be scheduled every two to three months until progress is stable and predictable. Repetition of the medicine will depend on the type of dosing being used. Your homeopath will determine the frequency of dosing based on your child's response to the medicine. Steady improvement should occur with proper repetition of the medicine in the correct strength or potency. Very positive changes take place rapidly in some cases, but more slowly in others. The *trend* of improvement is more important than the pace. The most profound effects in homeopathy occur over months and years, as the state of body and mind that created the imbalance is reduced or eliminated. With regular treatment, improvements will likely continue and stabilize. This stabilization process occurs over one to two years. Patients who leave treatment before they are stable may lose some, or all, of the benefits they have gained. Gradually, the frequency of visits will be reduced until the desired treatment goals are met.

What to Expect from Homeopathic Treatment of ASD

In our experience, the following list contains reasonable expectations for a child with ASD. If your child is more impaired, his progress may be slower or more limited. Having said that, we have worked with some children on the less-able end of the continuum who exhibit spectacular responses to homeopathic treatment!

Some ASD symptoms respond more readily to

homeopathy than others. The list below details our own experience in treating ASD kids. Each child is different, but these categories can give you a general sense of your child's prognosis:

Highly Likely to Improve with Homeopathic Treatment:
* restlessness
* mood changes
* impulsivity
* concentration difficulties
* school performance
* angry outbursts
* oppositional behavior
* socially inappropriate behavior
* most physical complaints
* hypersensitivity
* confidence and self-esteem issues
* awkwardness in interpersonal relationships
* social isolation
* ability to make friends
* obsessive behavior
* inability to participate in team sports

Will Probably Get Better with Homeopathic Treatment:
* perseveration
* eye contact
* learning disabilities
* pickiness
* self-stimulatory behavior
* tics
* hyperfocus on special interests
* encopresis (bowel impaction)
* bedwetting
* echolalia

You May Possibly See Changes with Homeopathic Treatment:
• developmental delays
• "pedantic" speech
• lack of empathy
• inability to speak

How Do I Find a Competent Homeopath?

Investigate the training and experience of any prospective homeopath. Inquire about her level of experience in treating chronic, pediatric and psychiatric conditions, and specifically ASD. Some practitioners have met certain standards, such as naturopathic doctors who are board certified by the Homeopathic Academy of Naturopathic Physicians (HANP), medical doctors who hold the certification of D.Ht., or those who have passed the examinations of the Council on Homeopathic Certification (CHC) or the North American Society of Homeopaths (NASH). These organizations and others such as the National Center for Homeopathy maintain referral lists, which may be helpful for finding a homeopath in your area. (See the Appendix for referral sources.)

Using Homeopathy and Conventional Medicine Together

Some parents choose to use both homeopathic and conventional medication concurrently. The two forms of treatment may be complementary and work together well. It is unlikely that the homeopathic medicine will interfere with the conventional treatment, but sometimes the prescription drug does impact the homeopathic medicine. If this occurs, we simply repeat the homeopathic medicine or adjust the dosage until the problem is resolved. If we are unable to find a resolution, we may recommend choosing between conventional and homeopathic treatment in the best interests of your child. Many children with ASD are already being treated conventionally with pharmaceutical medications when they begin homeopathic treatment. As naturopathic physicians, it is not within our scope of practice to discontinue a medication prescribed by another physician. *If, as a parent, you want to stop or decrease the dosage of your child's psychiatric or another prescription medication, you should consult with your child's prescribing physician. Abruptly discontinuing some medications is inadvisable and can be dangerous.*

At the beginning of treatment, we recommend against changing the currently prescribed conventional medicine. We also recommend against beginning any new interventions at the same time, conventional or alternative. It is best to keep the process as clear and simple as possible to avoid confusion for both the conventional and the homeopathic practitioners.

The main difficulty with using both kinds of medication together is determining which medicine is producing which results or side effects. This can be complex, especially if the patient is receiving a number of conventional medications at the same time, each with their own side effects and possible drug interactions. To achieve the best possible results with homeopathy, we have to be able to see the actual symptoms of the person, as well as any changes as they occur. If these symptoms or changes are masked by a psychiatric medicine, it may be difficult to know what is happening with homeopathic treatment, and similarly, the conventional doctor may attribute the success of the homeopathy to the pharmaceutical drugs.

Often, since homeopathy treats the whole child, the homeopathic medicine will produce positive changes that the conventional medications do not address, confirming that it is indeed working along with the other treatment. If your goal is to replace the conventional medications your child is now taking, or to decrease the dosage or number of different medications, you may want to ask your physician about doing so *before* beginning homeopathic treatment.

What If My Doctor Does Not Believe in Homeopathy?

Some parents find that seeking treatment in both medical worlds can be tricky, unless their conventional physician is open-minded enough to at least consider homeopathy as a viable treatment option. Some physicians refuse to work with parents who are also having their child treated homeopathically. Remember, you always have a choice regarding what type of treatment your child receives. If you wish to keep a foot in both worlds, you may wish to do what is necessary to find an open-minded physician to care for your child. Ideally your homeopath and conventional physician can work hand in hand for the benefit of your child.

Gradually, as more conventional medical doctors are learning about and using homeopathy, old prejudices are beginning to change. Some open-minded physicians are referring their unsolvable or baffling cases to homeopaths, or are incorporating homeopathy into their own practices. Many conventional medical students are eager to learn about homeopathy, as well as other forms of alternative medicine and nutrition. When choosing a homeopath, however, we advise finding a practitioner soundly trained in the field with at least several years of practice and an active continuing education program, rather than a conventional practitioner who is just dipping his feet into the waters of complementary or homeopathic medicine.

What to Avoid While Being Treated with Homeopathy

Certain substances and influences interfere with the action of a homeopathic medicine, a situation called *antidoting*. When this happens, it is usually necessary to repeat the homeopathic medicine in whatever dose is being currently prescribed. Once repeated, progress is usually reestablished and symptoms once again diminish or disappear. Occasionally, the potency of the medicine will need to be changed to obtain optimal results.

Antidoting is a controversial subject. Many homeopaths, ourselves included, observe that the action of homeopathic medicines can be interrupted by some substances—eucalyptus, camphor, menthol, tea tree oil, and coffee among them—or by the use of recreational drugs or electric blankets. Whether these factors are disruptive appears to be dependent upon the sensitivity of the individual child. Since different homeopaths have varying attitudes towards antidoting, rely on your own practitioner's recommendations. In any case, if the medicine that was working well for your child seems to stop working, regardless if there was any identifiable reason, let your homeopath know right away.

Conventional and other natural therapies, allergens, and foods to which a child is sensitive are not usually problematic, but sometimes can cause a relapse of symptoms. Therapeutic ultrasound, ultrasonic dental cleaning, and magnetic resonance imaging (MRI) may interfere with homeopathic treatment in some cases. If these are likely to be ongoing issues, or if you notice a change in the action of your child's homeopathic medicine after receiving such a treatment, consult with your homeopath. Acute childhood illnesses have also been known to interrupt the action of previously well-acting homeopathic medicines and may require a repetition of the previous medicine or the prescription of a different one that specifically addresses the acute symptom picture. Again, this response will vary with the individual.

How You Can Assist the Homeopathic Process

❧ *Provide your homeopath with thorough and honest information*
Withholding information for whatever reason may interfere with successful homeopathic treatment. Rest assured that your child's homeopathic medical records are confidential unless you sign a release to allow access by a third party.

❧ *Follow up with appointments at intervals recommended by your homeopath*
In large part, the ultimate success of your child's treatment depends on its continuity and consistency.

❧ *Inform you homeopath of significant changes in your child's life*
Important events in the family, academic progress, parental divorce or remarriage, moving, changing schools, making friends, or the death of a beloved pet are all worth sharing with your homeopath.

Homeopathy Is Not for Every Child

Not every youngster is a good candidate for homeopathic treatment. Some situations that can prevent successful treatment include:

❦ *Children who are resistant to treatment*
Some rebellious children, particularly adolescents, may try to sabotage homeopathic or other treatments out of opposition to their parents' wishes. They may miss appointments, refuse to talk to the practitioner, hide information such as drug use, refuse to take the medicine, or intentionally come into contact with substances that antidote it. Savvy homeopaths can sometimes salvage the therapeutic relationship with a heart-to-heart talk with the adolescent.

❦ *Parents who can't agree on treatment*
Ideally, both parents need to agree to having their child treated homeopathically, and be willing to give it a chance for at least a year. When one parent is opposed, or the parents are separated or divorced, difficulties in following through with treatment may arise. These problems are not insurmountable, but need to be dealt with if treatment is to work. If you think your child's other parent will be uncooperative with treatment (or will even deliberately sabotage it!), or if there are custody issues that will affect continuity of treatment, advise your homeopath.

❦ *Children who need institutional care*
Some children and adolescents with ASD are so difficult to manage that they need institutional placement or incarceration rather than outpatient treatment. We have successfully treated children in such settings, but the conditions are far from optimal.

Avoid the Temptation to Treat Your ASD Child with Homeopathy Yourself

As you read the case studies in this book, you may find one or two cases that closely resemble your child. You may be tempted to find the medicine that we gave and treat your child yourself. Don't even think about it!

While it is possible to treat yourself and your family for many first-aid conditions and acute minor illnesses yourself (see our book, *Homeopathic Self-Care*), ASD is *not* an acute condition, but rather a complex, chronic imbalance. It takes a competent, well-trained homeopath to prescribe for these cases. Only after years of homeopathic study and practice is it possible to understand symptoms, behavior, and homeopathic medicines well enough to match the correct homeopathic medicine to the child.

Even if you *were* to find the correct medicine, it takes experience to bring each case to a successful conclusion. Let your homeopath do his work. If you needed surgery, you wouldn't just get a book and a scalpel and start cutting! Your homeopath has the same level of experience in his field as a surgeon. Don't shortchange yourself or your child. Find a well-trained, experienced homeopath, and commit yourself to the full treatment process.

Does Homeopathic Treatment Feel Right for my ASD Child?

Parents frequently know that homeopathy is right for their children the moment they read the case histories (See Part Three). The children in this book may bear an uncanny resemblance to your own youngster. That feeling of "I am not alone" can be very comforting to parents who have been struggling for years with the isolation

ASD so frequently creates for families. Reading about how homeopathy has helped similar children provides hope that your child, too, may be helped. However, just because your child resembles one of the children whose case histories appear in this book, it does not mean he will need the same homeopathic medicine.

5

What Parents Say
Living With ASD Before and After Homeopathy

It is one thing for *us*, as homeopaths, to tell you how effective our medicine can be for many children with AS. We also want you to hear firsthand from parents whose kids have experienced the benefits of homeopathy.

As part of our research for this book, a number of the parents whose children's cases appear in chapters 6-10, were kind enough to answer the following questions:

1. What was your experience in the homeopathic interview?
2. If your child is old enough, what was the interview like for her?
3. What were your expectations regarding homeopathic treatment?
4. What changes have you seen in your child?
5. How has homeopathic treatment impacted your family?
6. What would you like to tell other parents of children similar to yours about homeopathy?

From their answers, we have excerpted the material that we thought would help you the most to decide whether homeopathy might be of benefit for *your* child.

(The names used for the children in this chapter, while fictitious, will be used again in chapters six through ten to refer to the same children.)

Jimmy

We were surprised that the initial appointment was so lengthy. And that Dr. Reichenberg-Ullman had actually worked with other children like Jimmy. She suggested that a diagnosis of Semantic Pragmatic Disorder might fit him better than Asperger Syndrome. When I looked it up on the web, it seemed very accurate for him. The fact that she seemed to have quite a bit of experience with kids like Jimmy was comforting. Jimmy was actually looking forward to meeting the doctor. His brother, also diagnosed with AS, had done so well under her care that Jimmy asked to see her, too. He told me he 'wanted to get going' himself.

I had resisted the idea of homeopathy. With two kids who had struggled with the condition for years, I knew (or thought) there were no quick cures. But, as a Special Education teacher myself, I met a mother whose son had made considerable progress by going to Dr. Reichenberg-Ullman. When I was ready (desperate), I took one of my sons to see her. I was a little ashamed to be going in for one of those 'last hope' treatments. Then I read one of their books and could hardly wait to get started.

Jimmy is very different than when we first took him to Dr. Reichenberg-Ullman. He was so depressed that we wondered about putting him on antidepressants. This year everyone around him comments on how much happier and more outgoing he is with other children and adults. It is fascinating, because he continues to improve even more. Jimmy is much more focused, cares about getting his schoolwork done for the first time, is much more even-tempered, and is able to respond when we ask him to do chores. He even often, though not always, keeps his room clean. Jimmy is very involved in sports and is doing well in them. An active Boy Scout, he is quite popular in the troop. Jimmy is quite the normal kid. Our son is also concerned with doing the right thing, and will stick his neck out with the other kids more than before. I especially like that he has more of a sense of humor. The boy just seems more relaxed.

I do believe that this treatment will be the means to my two sons living successful, independent lives. Their progress has motivated me to have treatment myself. I have also found it to be very helpful. I didn't realize how much time I spent being depressed and angry until I wasn't anymore. Homeopathy for me has helped me to appreciate the continued improvements in the boys as well as to find my own healing. It is hard to believe that a ten-dollar medicine could make such a positive difference months and months after taking it. I think we are all more hopeful. We were so impressed that our whole family is now being treated with homeopathy.

I know the whole process can seem expensive, but nothing we have ever done has been so worthwhile for our kids. While we took our second son to speech therapy for years, he was actually able to finally speak intelligibly once he received a homeopathic remedy. But it doesn't necessarily happen quickly. It took our second son several visits to find the right remedy, but this has been a life-changing experience for all of us. We have healing that we have never had before. We also have hope for the future.

I understand that homeopathy doesn't work for everyone, but it has been very successful for us. As a special education teacher, my dream would be for all of my children with Asperger's to have the option of homeopathic treatment. I think the results would be phenomenal.

Jai

Three months prior to his third birthday, I knew Jai was on his way to some sort of diagnosis. I didn't know what was wrong with him, but I, and other people, just knew that he was not a normal two-year-old boy. Something was not right. I started him on the Feingold Program at this time, and eliminated all artificial colors and preservatives from his diet. Jai's disposition changed rapidly. I saw him happily singing and hugging for the first time in a very long time. If he ate anything he had a sensitivity to, then a very miserable child emerged again. I knew he could not live the rest of his life like this. Changing his diet made a lot of symptoms disappear, but I knew there had to be a reason beyond food sensitivities that was causing such a young child to have such a horrible disposition. Through the advice of a mom whose child was helped by homeopathy, I decided to make an appointment.

In our first telephone interview with Dr. Luepker, we spent two hours talking about Jai from head to toe, inside and out. We started with him in the womb and worked our way up to the present time. Jai was too young to talk to the doctor him-

self, but Dr. Luepker knew what questions to ask in order to figure out what was going on with him. It was kind of amazing to spend two hours with a doctor who was asking for more information about all the little things that everyone else just patted you on the head for, and sent you on your way thinking that you were crazy. It's not easy for a mom to view her child as not normal, especially when everyone else wants to blame you for not parenting properly.

Because of knowing another mom whose child was helped with homeopathy, I expected that within two years Jai's food sensitivities would be gone, just like her son's. I was surprised when, within a year of starting his treatment, Jai was able to eat almost any food without having reactions. I knew we were getting to the root of his problems with homeopathy. Jai is no longer hyperactive. He doesn't have temper tantrums. Our son is one of the most affectionate four-year olds I know. Jai doesn't let any of us leave the house without giving him hugs and kisses. He'd cuddle on our laps and read books for hours if he could. Although still hesitant in showing loving affection to people outside the home, Jai no longer growls and snarls at people who talk to him. Still a shy child, he does try more and more to speak to people when spoken to. Jai is also much more sensitive to younger children, realizing the need to care for them.

Thanks to homeopathy, we see a normal child before us. Jai will be able to function in a normal classroom, without sticking out like a sore thumb. Other people don't complain about his discipline problems anymore. I knew I would never medicate my son, no matter what it took. By the grace of God, homeopathy has given Jai the freedom to eat what the other kids eat at birthday parties, and the freedom to run and play like other boys his age, instead of standing on the sidelines watching the fun and not having any himself. Homeopathy gets to the root of the problem instead of just covering up the symptoms like medication does. One of the best gifts a parent can give a child is to make sure they are the healthiest they can be, so they can reach their fullest potential in whatever they do. Homeopathy can achieve this without side effects. Now that Jai has done so wonderfully, I have just begun to be treated myself.

Chris

Dr. Reichenberg-Ullman asked tons of questions about our son that were unlike any asked by an MD She got very specific about daily habits, emotions, fears, dreams, and quirks. She even asked what makes our son special or different from anyone else. Since our son had received homeopathic care before... all the obvious possibilities had been tried already. Our main expectation was to be able to live with him more comfortably, and to try to keep him in mainstream schools.

Chris was six, heading into first grade, and he was completely capable of being interviewed. However, when the doctor tried to videotape him, she mostly got footage of the empty chair. Sitting was impossible. He moved constantly and was not very coherent in his answers the first time. Chris was also very obsessive-compulsive at this point, washing his hands forty to sixty times a day. He kept touching things all over the office, with both hands an equal number of times.

Within a couple of days after taking the first medicine Dr. R. prescribed, the hand washing stopped, as did Chris' continual rhyming. When he started first grade, his teacher told us she saw no difference between him and any other first grader.

We were already familiar with the changes possible with homeopathy, but were unprepared for the large-scale transformation of our son. He had been thrown out of two daycares as an infant and almost expelled several times from kindergarten. Ever since the first-grade, the positive changes have persisted. His fifth-grade teacher considers him one of the best students and nicest kids in the class.

Chris started making friends in the first grade, right after we took him to see Dr. R., but rarely had play dates. Now he does fairly well keeping up socially with the kids in his class, though he still has some playground issues. Chris has a group of kids he considers friends, but no one he considers his best friend. He's still not entirely sure of the motives of the other boys who seem to be teasing him.

One teacher with AS experience related to me that Chris looks completely normal in a group of kids. He now has much more fluid, normal-looking facial expressions and speaks more flowingly, rather than the choppier, random speech pattern he had previously. We've also seen a big change in his writing style. Chris' hypersensitivity has also calmed greatly in many respects, though he still has some hearing issues.

He is much easier to live with. Random noises are less frequent. Although still fairly talkative, he can calm himself down. Much less fearful, our son has a significantly better grasp of fantasy versus reality. We went camping last summer several times without his being afraid of bugs, darkness, snakes, and sharks. Chris' diet has widened considerably and he handles unfamiliar tastes and textures much more easily. Most of all, he has become much more empathetic and understanding of other people's feelings. Oh, yes, he sleeps now! A huge improvement to all of our lives!

I would like to tell any other parents at their wits' end that there truly is hope. It may take a few remedy trials, but this therapy reaches into the souls and unties knots, allowing the true self to emerge. I felt like such a failure as a mother before Chris was treated, and society reinforced that feeling. Our whole family felt isolated and frazzled most of the time. This medicine is allowing Chris to develop like a normal child who, no doubt, will grow into an amazing adult.

This has changed all our lives, by far, for the better. We can have a social life, drive in the car for more than thirty minutes, and eat dinner together— all eating the same thing! We don't have to apologize to teachers or other parents anymore for Chris' behavior. We can buy pants with buttons and zippers rather than just soft sweatpants. We look forward to seeing him through school and career successfully and, finally, we have a loving, demonstrative, intelligent, funny son. Whew!!

Gina

The interview was long and thorough. Dr. Ullman asked many questions, probing in a good way, drawing out the information he needed. I was able to bring all of my observations and concerns into the interview. I knew what to expect from discussions on the Feingold bulletin board and had prepared pages of notes. The interview was give and take. Dr. Ullman questioned, listened, asked for more details or clarification, and then questioned again.

My daughter was six years old when we had our initial interview with Dr. Ullman. We had sought out homeopathic treatment for our daughter after more than two years on stage one of the Feingold Program. We were not seeing the strides in her that we had expected in regarding salicylate sensitivity, environmental sensitivities, hyperactivity, and bizarre behaviors, that would eventually allow us to move to stage two. Gina did participate in the interview process, taking a turn after I had spoken for quite a while. She was actually eager to talk to Dr. Ullman and to answer his questions, especially enjoying all the attention she was given.

Over the past year and a half of homeopathic care, our daughter has become reachable. Now able to respond to correction, she is much more in the 'here and now'. Before we saw Dr. Ullman, there appeared to be no bond between us, no connection. Now she is affectionate (she was not at all before). Gina used to not even be able to hold a crayon and now she loves art. And she doesn't torment the cat anymore.

Try it! The results are surprising, though sometimes slow and subtle. It is non-invasive. A welcome contrast to conventional medicine.

Conner

I was a little surprised at the depth and background of questions. Things I hadn't really thought about, like birth experience and food likes or dislikes came up. As I learned more about homeopathy, I came to understand how important this deep background information was to his case. I was impressed at how, for the first time in six years of saying 'something is not right with my son' to medical professionals, I felt listened to, and it was clear that Dr. Reichenberg thought my observations had validity. It was like a light coming on, after struggling uphill in the dark for years.

An Internet acquaintance from the Feingold Bulletin Board, whose son exhibited behaviors and symptoms similar to my son's, had seen Dr. Ullman and been very pleased with the results. I was hoping for anything that might help my family lead something resembling a normal life.

I knew it could take a while, and that the 'whole person' approach to wellness, while deep, might be subtle. That has proved to be our experience. It took several near-misses for us to find the correct remedy, but when we did, the results were SO dramatic that his teacher, unaware we were seeing a homeopathic doctor said, 'He's like a different kid.' When you get the right homeopathic medicine, you will know.

When my son began homeopathic treatment at age six, he would not sleep alone, rarely slept through the night, and had violent meltdown rages at least twice a week. The outbursts were usually over something as trivial as having to change his shirt, or not getting his favorite color cup. The contrast is remarkable.

Conner recently had his first tantrum in almost nine months, and it was minor by the 'bad old days' standard. He walks himself to and from school, bathes himself, dresses himself, makes his own lunch, and happily stays home alone for short periods. Conner didn't read at all until the very end of second grade. Shortly after finally finding the correct remedy, he began to read. By September, when he was tested again for school, he was reading at the fourth grade level. By the following May, one year after beginning to read, he was reading at a seventh grade level and had been invited to bring his writing to a regional young writer's conference. Conner tests above grade level in most areas now, and was in danger of losing his IEP! Things are MUCH calmer, and I'm more able to do the real fun work of parenting rather than just fighting fires all the time.

What I see, more than anything, is that homeopathy has been a tool for my son to gain control over his sensory input and his reaction to 'overload.' With that tool, he can turn his attention to other things instead of just trying to process the flicker of the fluorescent lights and the texture of the carpet. The change has been remarkable for all of us!

I would say to any parent of an AS child: 'Try homeopathy, and really commit to really making it work'. Most of us have a lot of experience with 'quick-fix' medicine (and food, and relationships, and...) Homeopathy will not work that way. When you do find the right remedy, the initial response may be dramatic, but the real, deep change will take some time. It may not work for everyone. In his case, the eventual results have pretty clearly justified the trouble and expense. If you spend the money and show the results now, some kid in twenty years will be able to get homeopathic treatment for autism covered by insurance. Think of yourself as a pioneer.

Noah

We were very excited to have been able to make an appointment with Dr. Ullman. We live in the U.K. and had first considered homeopathy for Noah after reading their book, Ritalin-Free Kids. *We found a good homeopath in England, but were still very keen to see Dr. Bob as we knew he specialized in children with behavioral difficulties. We had very positive expectations that Dr. Bob could make a difference to our son, and we were thrilled with the changes that we saw in our son after homeopathic treatment.*

We had begun to despair about Noah at the time we started the homeopathy. Noah had already made great progress with his autism through the Son-Rise program of the Option Institute, moving from being non-verbal to verbal with temper tantrums. His progress, however, had stalled for some time, and he had even regressed. Seldom interactive, Noah was showing less eye contact and talked incessantly of numbers.

The interview was very thorough, and we felt reassured by the depth and length of the visit, which covered Noah's life from the beginning. So often with general practitioners, we have felt that we do not get the opportunity to mention all the background we believe might be relevant

Very soon after taking the Silica, *we saw amazing improvements in Noah. The obsession with numbers abated, and he became more interactive and open to learning. Noah has continued to make progress, and we have seen improvements after each dose of the remedy. Now in a mainstream school, he is doing very well academically and plays appropriately with other children on the playground. We still have work to do with him, but he is steadily progressing.*

We would urge any parent of an autistic child or a child with behavioral problems to try homeopathy. You have everything to gain and nothing to lose.

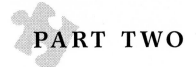

PART TWO

Actual Cases of Children on the Autism Spectrum

6

Awkward and Alienated
Human Behavior Does Not Compute

Parents confide in us with great frequency that their children are excluded or ostracized by their peers for being different. The youngster is the only one in her class not invited to birthday parties. Play date invitations are not reciprocated. She is always chosen last for sports teams.

Parents, naturally, have high hopes for their children's happiness, which includes interactive play and mutual friendships. How heartbreaking to learn that your child eats lunch by herself day after day, or, even worse, that her peers move to another table when she sits down to join them. Or to discover that she is being bullied or taunted by the "popular girls" or called "weird" just for being herself.

Some kids with ASD appear to be oblivious to the scorn and derision. Other youngsters avoid the subject entirely, insisting that they do have friends, even though it is not the case. A recent front-page story in our local newspaper documented the tragic experience of an adolescent with AS who was unsuccessful at making any friends. The isolation was so painful that he eventually took his own life. At the funeral, attended by a patient of ours who herself has two sons with AS, the mom bravely displayed photos portraying the life, cut prematurely short, of her deceased son. Her mission, she explained, was to appreciate the precious child that her family knew rather than the boy who never fit in with the crowd. The mourners were deeply moved by the poignant message. The first thing parents often confide in us is, "My child is just different." Different from siblings, peers, and classmates, friends, extended family members. Among any age group, individuals who stand out run the risk of ostracism. Put an unusual child into a group of children or adolescents, and the chances of her being singled out and made fun of are high. At an age when youngsters are just learning the meaning of friendship and trust, children with ASD may not have even one person to call a real friend.

A child with ASD may display strange gestures, be unable to maintain eye contact, and exhibit a stiff, formal affect. Such kids rarely stand a chance of peer acceptance. Some learn to take on good enough "protective coloration" (as one AS adult that we know calls it) to go unnoticed, but that's not really belonging to a group. If a child's special ability is something other children find useful (like rattling off sports statistics), she may manage to become something of a "mascot," but probably will not really fit in.

Assuming your child is not successful at disappearing, she is likely to stand out among any group of peers. You can hope she is oblivious to social ostracism, has some endearing feature that her peers can appreciate, or that her class is filled with nice, tolerant kids rather than callous bullies. In most cases, social skills training will be needed throughout your child's school years, to teach her the rudiments and subtleties of social behavior. We find that homeopathic treatment can be a great boon to increasing social acceptance of children with ASD. You may be surprised to learn that homeopathy can actually change how other youngsters respond to your child, but it is true.

Alan: Oblivious to Social Cues

Alan, age seven, had been formally diagnosed with AS. The child had suffered an intractable nine-month bout of hives following an MMR immunization. This history, in addition to chronic rectal itching and diarrhea, had prompted another homeopath to prescribe *Sulphur*, which produced a significant overall improvement lasting only a week. It was Alan's social and behavioral challenges that led his mother, Pam, to seek out our care.

Pam described her son as "so much in his own world" that he could barely carry on a conversation. Even when Alan did manage to hold up his end of a dialogue, others dismissed his comments as irrelevant and ignored him. Social cues went right over Alan's head. He rarely maintained eye contact with those who spoke to him. When Alan initiated a discussion, he tended to monopolize the conversation, without noticing whether the other person was actually listening. The youngster had quite a talent for singing and an excellent memory for tunes and lyrics. He could ramble for hours about his favorite song or computer game until his listener's eyes glazed over. Even then, he hadn't a clue that the other person was bored.

One disturbing topic of conversation was Alan's frequent references to hurting or killing people. Though many children make these types of threats idly, the rash of school shootings at the time worried the adults who knew about them. They became even more concerned when, instead of merely squabbling with his brother, Alan wrapped a radio cord tightly around his neck.

Alan's family and teachers described the boy as "naïve, gullible, and literal." A shy child, Alan had the habit of lowering his head or hiding behind his mother in new situations. The youngster exhibited a number of socially unacceptable behaviors, including chewing, touching others, biting his nails, and pacing. He also had the curious habit of taking three steps to the right, turning to the left, then repeating the sequence over and over. Alan was clumsy on the soccer field and seemed to lack any understanding of the rules of the game. It was not that he was universally uncoordinated. In fact, the boy was an avid and agile climber. But, when asked to undertake a particular physical task, such as kicking a ball, his coordination seemed to disappear.

Alan's peers were keenly aware of his social deficits and referred to him as "weird." They enjoyed razzing him or getting him to say and do embarrassing things. Alan was fascinated by computers, though his grasp of how they worked was more elementary than he led others to believe. His overly eager patter about the computer game of the day, and anything related to technology, were perceived by others as badgering. When he approached them, they headed in the opposite direction. Alan's apparent lack of empathy only exacerbated the problem. If another child were hurt or in trouble, he appeared unconcerned and interested only in his own needs.

Alan's voice was annoyingly loud, even in his calmest moments. When the youngster became upset, he shrieked at the top of his lungs—so piercingly that the rest of the family covered their ears. Whenever his parents engaged in conversation with each other, Alan found some reason to wrest their attention in order to address his seemingly urgent need. If they argued, the boy intervened, yelling for them to stop.

During the pregnancy, Pam had suffered considerable insecurity. She and her husband engaged in ongoing verbal battles. Pam experienced a great fear of abandonment, and felt threatened by the least suggestion of being ignored by her husband. It did not help matters that Alan's father was leery of commitment. One more baby on the way made him think seriously about leaving the marriage. Pam had been previously left after being impregnated by another man, and worried constantly that it could happen again. We mention these family dynamics, even during the pregnancy, because they can play a significant role in the symptoms that a child develops.

Exceptional Features

 Alan exhibited a number of common characteristics of AS: difficulty with social cues and interactions; fixation on computers, Nintendo and technology (though this characteristic alone is a common contemporary generational feature); lack of eye contact; self-absorption; and lack of interest in other peer activities such as sports. Alan's grand passion for computers and technology were his constant topic of conversation, causing him to be perceived as pushy and opinionated, and, therefore, alienating potential friends.

Alan had symptoms of two common homeopathic medicines, *Baryta carbonica* (barium carbonate) and *Sulphur* (sulfur). Children who need *Baryta carbonica* are known for being developmentally or academically delayed, shy, and dependent. Their tendency towards awkwardness and immaturity leads others to tease and laugh at them. The derision leads them to keep to themselves, often fading into the woodwork in order to avoid calling further attention to themselves. *Sulphur* patients, on the other hand, are strongly opinionated and enjoy engaging in lively debate or pontificating on their favorite subjects, seeming to care little about the interests and feelings of others. The one area of sensitivity to which those needing *Sulphur* are prone is to criticism, insults, or scorn. These youngsters typically display a strong interest in, and talent for, mechanical and technological pursuits. They often love to take objects apart in order to learn how they work. Itchy rashes, hives, and rectal itching, previous symptoms of Alan, are common to those needing Sulphur.

When a patient exhibits characteristics of two different homeopathic medicines made from minerals, the mineral salt containing both components is indicated. In this case, the medicine was *Baryta sulphuricum* (barium sulfate). In the homeopathic literature, the symptom "fear of conversation" is attributed to those needing this medicine. It is of interest in this case given Alan's inability to engage in dialogue rather than monologue. We have used this symptom to choose *Baryta sulphuricum* in other cases in which, like in Alan's, there was a marked deficit in conversational ability.

Greater Empathy and Socialization
Alan's initial response to the first two doses of *Baryta sulphuricum* was promising. At the two-month follow-up appointment, Pam described him as more aware and less "in his own world." He was better able to socialize with his peers, and he exhibited greater empathy and self-control. The episodes of unruly behavior had diminished. Alan's spelling improved and, for the first time, his academic performance fell within the guidelines of his Individualized Educational Program (IEP).

Over the next four months, Alan continued to improve academically, behaviorally, and socially. The quality of his schoolwork continued to progress, as did his appropriateness in the classroom. Alan's parents were pleasantly surprised that he had become demonstrably more caring for family members and peers. His shyness lessened. During the entire time he had experienced only one aggressive outburst, during which he threatened to cut people's heads off with a knife. Otherwise he was calmer and did not exhibit violent tendencies. Although friends were still elusive, Alan was quite a bit more capable of interacting with peers.

We gave Alan three doses of the *Baryta sulphuricum* over the course of a year, at this point, compared to the boy we first treated a year earlier, his mother called Alan "the perfect child." No longer aggressive or threatening, far calmer, no longer confined to his own world, Alan was, by and large, free of the behaviors other children considered strange. The boy was much more acceptable to his peers and was making progress socially. His interest in others had increased. He tended to "borrow" his brother's friends rather than making his own, and he still enjoyed showing off his knowledge to anyone who would listen. He was far more empathic than when we first met him, in fact, others commented on how kind he was to small children. Alan's teachers were impressed with how much of a difference homeopathy had made. Academically, he excelled in math, science and spelling, though writing was still challenging.

Alan has continued to need a dose of *Baryta sulphuricum* once or twice a year. The improvement in all areas continues. The child is now in a mainstream classroom and much more at ease socially. Alan's parents, family, and teachers are quite pleased.

Angie: The Girl Who Swore, Spat, and Barked

Angie, an eight-year-old redhead from Memphis, was diagnosed with ADHD when we first saw her. Although she was not diagnosed with AS at the time of our first visit, she was later formally diagnosed with AS. Angie had taken a variety of psychotropic medications by the time her parents consulted us. Ritalin didn't work, Adderall made her spacey and caused nightmares, and she became overly excitable on Wellbutrin. When we started treating Angie, she was taking Imipramine, which was supposed to "settle her down." An expert at pushing her mother's buttons, Angie purposely slammed doors, changed the wake-up setting on her mother's alarm clock, and engaged in many other intentionally provocative acts.

The child exhibited a number of inappropriate, socially unacceptable behaviors. She gave those around her the finger as she uttered the "F" word, not just occasionally, but one hundred or so times a day. As if this habit were not unusual enough, Angie immediately and profusely apologized after each of the behaviors. These outbursts alienated her from other children and adults alike, to the point of her being expelled from several daycare centers. Despite her constant outpouring of profanity, Angie refused to watch any television program that was violent in nature, even cartoons.

Born with clubbed feet and a lack of growth hormone, Angie received injections of Protropin six days a week. Despite a delay in her ability to sit up by herself (age two) and to walk (age four), she was quite bright. Yet, when faced with homework, she insisted, "I can't do it. It's too hard. I need help." Placed in a special education class because of her behavioral problems and social inappropriateness, Angie engaged with peers by either pinching them or shying away from them. Needless to say, none of the other children was inclined to be her friend. Angie had a passion for any type of map. So strong was this focus of interest that the child even requested a "Thomas Guide" for Christmas rather than toys or dolls.

Angie needed her mom right there with her to do anything—even to bathe or go to the bathroom—so much so that her mother described the two of them as "Siamese twins". She even banged on the bathroom door when her mom sought out a moment of privacy to relieve herself. The youngster exhibited an inordinate terror of tornadoes. During storm season, she asked her mother every night if a twister were on its way. Rain also frightened the child, prompting her to call her mom from school, if there were a storm, to remind her to drive home slowly. Angie feared animals, especially dogs, and had been bitten on the face by a dog at the age of three. Extremely sensitive to loud noises, she covered her ears if a loud truck passed by, or if there was a fire drill practice at school. The girl's mom had to provide the youngster with earplugs whenever she went to a movie. Angie also had a habit of twisting her hair and chewing on furry clothing, like velour. The child had never been a good sleeper, and she suffered from recurrent headaches.

When we began treating Angie, her parents decided to take her off the Wellbutrin and Imipramine, which made her symptom picture much clearer. Prior to taking the medications, she had a strange phobia of the reflections of shiny objects. Now the fear was much more intense. Angie avoided eating at the dinner table unless all the lights were turned off, due to the light reflected off several pictures on the table. Her parents noticed that all of the other frames that they had placed in their cabinets had been turned around so that they did not catch light.

Several other habits were more exaggerated without the medications. Angie swore and spit with great frequency. She spat all over the floor and at her babysitter. Another strange quirk was her tendency to lick other people's feet and arms. Her fear of dogs was intensified, and she had begun to make a weird, barking sound if her mother became upset with her. She avoided holding cats for fear they might scratch her. Also heightened was her dread of taking a bath. Since stopping the medications, whenever the lights in their swimming pool were illuminated, Angie ran out screaming, fearful that she would be sucked down the drain.

Angie's remorse immediately following her angry outbursts also became more prominent. She started to write letters of apology to her mom, perhaps twenty after each incident, in addition to her verbal regret. There would have been more, but her mother discouraged her excessive repentance.

Exceptional Features

 Although Angie did not carry the label of AS until a number of years after we first saw her, the lack of social appropriateness, obsession with particular notions, and developmental delays were suggestive of the diagnosis much earlier. As peculiar as Angie's symptoms may seem, there is a particular homeopathic medicine that fits her picture brilliantly. It is *Lyssin*, a nosode. The barking, spitting, and licking as well as her fear of dogs and bathing, her dislike of cats, and the history of being bitten by a dog fit the picture of *Lyssin* well. Even the fits of swearing and rage coupled with her apologetic nature appear in the homeopathic literature when describing this medicine. The symptoms of *Lyssin* may be brought on following a dog bite, or from repeated torment or harassment, both of which were true of Angie.

A Rapid and Dramatic Improvement

Five weeks after Angie took a single dose of *Lyssin*, her mother reported that the barking diminished considerably, as did the spitting and swearing. She now uttered a couple of bad words in a day compared to the hundred or so before taking the *Lyssin*. The reflections were no longer as much of a concern. The child's babysitter was amazed at how much better she behaved. Convincing

Angie to bathe was less of a battle. Her teachers found the improvement in her behavior at summer school to be nothing short of remarkable. One instructor even commented that she was actually beginning to be popular with her classmates. The licking and other obsessive tendencies were also diminished. Angie was still immature and continued to demand her mother's company constantly.

At her two-month follow-up telephone appointment, Angie's mother estimated that she was at least 75% better across the board. Her teachers continued to be amazed by the "new Angie". Not only did she now have friends at school, but she was busy with after-school play dates. The sensitivity to shiny glass continued to be better, as was the swearing. Bathing was no longer a dreaded event, and Angie no longer found it necessary to draft letters of apology *ad infinitum*. Angie needed nine doses of the *Lyssin* over the course of four years of treatment.

After a two year hiatus from treatment, we heard again from Angie's mother. Now fifteen years old, the teenager had been diagnosed with AS and she was experiencing headaches. The barking, sensitivity to reflections, and most of her other "odd behaviors" had not returned. She was, however, tapping her feet repetitively in class. Her obsession with maps remained to a lesser extent. They still excited her, but she no longer stared at them for three hours at a time as she did before she first saw us. The scratching and biting had never returned, although Angie still swore occasionally, mostly when her mother was not around. The mother attributed an 80-90% overall improvement to the homeopathy. Angie's main problem now, other than the headaches, was impulsivity. Dealing with other children and reading social cues was still difficult.

Since we had not treated Angie in two years, it was

important to ascertain whether she still needed the same medicine. It was probable, but a homeopath needs to remain ever open to the possibility that a different medicine may be indicated. Although Angie couldn't elaborate much on her headaches, she was able to describe how the other children picked on her and threw things at her on a daily basis. "They say I'm a loser and throw a sharp pencil at me. I feel sad and upset and want to really get 'em. But I just walk away. It's the same kids every day." When we inquired about her fears, Angie responded, "People picking on me. You know, the average things." We ended the interview by asking about her dreams. You guessed it: "People picking on me." Within two days of taking the *Lyssin*, Angie's headaches vanished.

William: The Boy Who Twisted Wire

William, fourteen years old, was brought to us, in large part, because of his academic and attitudinal problems. Paying attention in school was quite a challenge, as evidenced by below-average grades in language, math, and reading. His behavior deteriorated further when he ate dairy products. Melanie, William's mother, described her son as "narrow-minded, stubborn, rigid, and reluctant to venture into unfamiliar territory." When any request was made of William, his initial response was to scream, "No!" Twenty minutes later, he usually went ahead and completed the task.

In the third grade, William had taken Ritalin for a brief period of time. A thorough workup at age thirteen at the Mayo Clinic resulted in the diagnoses of AS, ADHD, and LD. The specialists concluded William ranked far behind his peers developmentally, despite his impressively articulate speech. Testing at the Pfeiffer

Institute had shown William to have an elevated copper/zinc ratio, leading to an extensive regimen of nutritional supplements over the previous four years.

During the interview William, was eager to speak for himself. The young man spoke slowly, seriously and ponderously—far more so than a typical teenager. Though William's affect was flat, and it was difficult to get him excited about anything, he expressed himself very adeptly. William's first words immediately caught our attention.

> *I bend and twist wire if I am bored. While I twist, I daydream about the future, what I'll do after college, stuff I saw before, and scenes from movies. I put my daydreaming on cruise control. My image of myself is 'the kid who twists the wire.' Twisting takes the edge off of being bored.*

A Highly Articulate Young Man

Melanie was concerned about her son's ongoing anxiety and recurrent episodes of anger. William became easily annoyed at little things, like his toddler cousins throwing fits, or his sister borrowing his DVDs and not returning them. Every now and then, the angry outburst became more intense, during which time William shouted and refused to obey his parents.

When asked about his fears, William was very articulate:

> *I hate spiders! They crawl on my skin. I hate snakes, too. Bats are really ugly and scary. They are creatures of the night. I hate great white sharks. They are scary and have yellow chunks of flesh hanging from their teeth. I don't like the idea of the speed of pain. I'm even afraid of a needle's prick. I hate needles. I even hate the idea of being stabbed with a*

needle. I freak out during a blood draw. Needles don't agree with me and I don't like them. I would never get a body part pierced. I had ingrown toenails and I really did not like the burning pain I felt during the surgery.

When we broached the subject of school, William launched into a tirade about his intensely dislike of a particular teacher.

In seventh grade I was very angry. My special-ed math teacher drove me over the edge. She was fat, mean, and really, really ugly. She yelled a lot. I suffered through the year. I'd come home tired, stressed, or upset about something. She was bossy, snotty, and had no patience. People are there in special-ed class because they don't get it. I guess my bad attitude prevented me from getting much out of the class.

"Oddball" Interests

When asked about hobbies or special interests, William elaborated, "I really like old movies, but my friends don't. I try to be socially acceptable, but it feels funny. I particularly like old horror movies like *Frankenstein*. I own 200 movies and 56 DVDs. I like thrillers. They are intense, exciting, and cool. My taste in movies is oddball."

"Oddball" was an apt description of how William perceived himself before receiving homeopathic treatment:

I have a lot of socially unacceptable things in my head. I'm not cool enough or social enough for those kids. All the girls started this 'William has cooties' thing, just like little kids. My social skills definitely

need work. I don't feel good enough to step into con-
versations. I scramble in my mind for things to say
without looking like a complete idiot. Sometimes I
talk about things that are above them. Or I decide
to not talk and just keep quiet.

I'm known as being kind of unsocial. I listen to
the preps to see what kinds of things they say. It used
to be worse. At least now I can strike up a conver-
sation. My pace is fast and slow. Fast and slow. I
won't be rushed by anybody if I'm not in the mood.
My mom says I don't know when to stop or start. If
I have one problem left and it is time to go, I have
to do it. I didn't start when she said to because I was
daydreaming.

My parents, my sister, and I fight a lot. My
mom is happy and jolly, I'm more moody and a not-
smiling-a-lot person. I'm very narrow-minded and
lazy. I don't want to do a lot of things, like read a
big book. I do like to work at my grandmother's
store. It's really huge, not boring like home. I have
trouble making decisions about what I want, like
what CD to buy. Should I just grab one and go or
spend two hours choosing? My dad is like that. He
sits back and thinks about things a long time.

Exceptional Features

 Like many children with AS, William was lacking in social skills and considered an "oddball"
not only by his own estimation, but by his peers
as well. Additionally, he had difficulty making
conversation. His mannerisms were stiff and his speech
ponderous. He willingly admitted that he was narrow-
minded, rigid, slow-paced, and had a negative attitude.
One of the most unusual features of the case was
William's description of his dreams. What a contrast for

such a seemingly non-reactive child to display such a strong sensitivity to needles and creatures that might bite him. We first prescribed *Baryta sulphuricum* (Barium sulfate), the same medicine that we gave to Alan in the preceding case. Though there was a definite improvement in some areas, we went on to find a better medicine for him, as we will explain later in the case.

More Acquaintances and a Real Friend
Melanie reported that he seemed calmer and happier within a week of taking the *Baryta sulphuricum*. No longer bouncing off the walls, his anger and anxiety had diminished. He began to initiate get-togethers with other teenagers. Interactions with his parents went more smoothly. For the first time, William broke into tears upon seeing his baby nephew fall down. This was a remarkable occurrence since his parents could count on one hand the number of times they had seen their son cry since the time he was a toddler. William admitted to us that he did have more friends.

Over the next few months, William progressed. Meltdowns were rare, grades steadily improved, and his interactions with his parents were better. The young man was invited to his first birthday party in several years, and attracted a friend who was calling regularly. William shared in the interview. "I've been studying more. I have one good friend and some acquaintances. I got in a fight today, though. I wrestled him down and punched him in the cranium. I can make conversation, but I'm not very good at it, and I can't talk to girls at all. I don't have any problem asking them to dance, though."

William continued to relax by twisting wire. His increased socialization, combined with his naiveté, had led him into some bad company and some less than optimal choices. When one of his new friends tried to commit suicide by taking an overdose of caffeine pills, William confided to his parents that he wished he would die or that the world would end in 2006, to his parents' alarm. With a bit of counseling from his parents, William eventually decided the friends he was hanging out with were the wrong crowd, and the suicidal feelings passed.

Further Improvement After Taking a Different Medicine

Despite William's improvement in a number of areas, we were not satisfied that we had found the best possible medicine for him. Six months into treatment, we restudied William's case and prescribed *Helleborus* (black hellebore). We chose this medicine primarily because of William's habit of staring off into space hypnotically while twisting wire, his slow pace, and strong sensitivity to pain as expressed in his dreams as well as his memory of the ingrown toenail surgery. Also characteristic of those needing *Helleborus* were William's withdrawn behavior, inability to comprehend, inattention, and inner anguish. Black hellebore is a member of the *Ranunculaceae* (buttercup family), which is indicated for children who are highly sensitive to various stimuli, including physical or emotional pain, clothing, noise, and the environment in general. Though slow and non-reactive externally, Williams' dreams showed a high degree of reactivity to pain, typical of those needing this medicine.

Over the next three months, William developed a greater ability to focus and, according to his teacher, was better equipped to take notes in class, to understand the subject matter, and to organize, complete, and turn in assignments. His sense of responsibility and ability to cooperate were also better, and his attitude had taken a much-needed turn towards optimism.

Despite glowing reports from those around him, William acknowledged little progress. What other people saw in him, he could not yet find in himself. We have found, over the years, that even when they have experienced a dramatic shift as a result of homeopathy, some children remain unaware of how much they have changed. This is one reason that we prefer to communicate with the parent(s) privately first during follow-up visits, before talking to the children without the parents being present.

A second dose of *Helleborus*, administered two months later, produced an even more significant result. William's reading level took a giant leap. In fact, in the course of one year, he progressed from a fourth- to an eleventh-grade level, thanks to a combination of the homeopathy and his LD program. Although this degree of improvement over such a short time may seem impossible, it is something we have seen in a number of children.

Never one to overestimate his own progress, William did begrudgingly admit to doing better with remembering his assignments and completing his schoolwork. He added that he was enjoying art classes and was considering becoming a tattoo artist, an interesting choice for someone who had been so upset by needles.

By his next appointment, six months after changing the medicine to *Helleborus,* his attitude was even sunnier compared to the original William. "Today is a good day," he shared, "I'm not angry or unhappy. I feel pretty good." This level of optimism, coming from Mr. Negativity, was impressive. The idea of a career as a tattoo artist had gone by the wayside due to lack of artistic ability. William had obtained his learner's permit to drive, another step in the direction of independence. Socially, his school year had ended on a positive note—he had gone to two punk rock concerts with friends, quite a victory for a teenager with AS.

During his two years of treatment, this youngster has made considerable progress in academics, social skills, mood, habits, and attitude. With continued treatment, it is likely that he will move even further towards a happier and more independent life.

Johanna: Bullied and on the Social Sidelines

Johanna came to us diagnosed with ADHD and on Ritalin, but you will notice that she displays a number of familiar features of ASD. As already mentioned, over 65% of children with ASD are first labeled with ADHD. Although Johanna had not gone through the full psychological assessment necessary to get a formal diagnosis of ASD, her diagnosis seemed clear to us. We debated about including cases that lack a full diagnostic workup. Although we do recommend a full diagnostic assessment to confirm the diagnosis, not all parents chose to go this route. Some of you, for a variety of reasons including financial limitations, will not be able to have your child undergo such an assessment. Ultimately, we decided to include a few children, including Johanna, in which the diagnosis seems clear to us despite the lack of psychological testing.

Johanna is a remarkable child and we believe that her case is well worth including. Fifth grade had gotten off to a rocky start for Johanna, and by mid-winter it hadn't become any easier. Johanna's mom aptly described her as "eccentric," and this became readily apparent as we interviewed her. The child's behaviors and interactions with other children either alienated or "grossed out" her peers, leaving her on the social sidelines. Like many children on the autism continuum, Johanna was an easy target for bullying and teasing because of her differences and her inability to pick up on her classmates' social cues. As a result, she would occasionally return home sad and bruised, following fights with the other children.

Johanna was clearly different. Her movements were a bit uncoordinated, her language overly formal, and her voice tone peculiar. Furthermore, she would laugh at inappropriate moments, and the quality of the laughter was unnerving and awkward. Her tongue protruded slightly when she spoke, which added to the peculiarity of her voice.

Her mom explained, "The school says that she invades her neighbor's space. She has no awareness of social boundaries or unspoken rules. She'll talk really loud, even when she's right in front of your face. Johanna doesn't seem to have a sense of normal conversation. Sometimes she'll start a conversation and neglect to give any context or reference for what she's saying."

Johanna frequently embroiled herself in fights or arguments with the other children, usually after being teased. Then, when a teacher would intervene, Johanna would get into trouble. "She is truthful to a fault!" her mom bemoaned. "When other kids provoke her to the point of defending herself, and she is caught, she will explain *everything* to the teacher, fully expecting him to believe her. When that does not happen, she doesn't feel listened to and becomes sad."

When Johanna first walked into our consultation room, she immediately began to investigate the room and its contents. "I'm curious about this room," she stated. "I like to know my surroundings. It makes me feel safer. And it's good to feel safe." She added, "At school, during recess, I feel unsafe. Other kids throw balls into my face and I can't participate in their games."

"I feel like no one likes me, not even my parents. People are on me. No one at school talks with me or wants to play with me. I feel sad a lot," Johanna explained. Her mom confirmed this, and was prompted, in part, to make an appointment with us because Johanna had been recently talking about suicide.

I Can Feel the Animal's Pain

Johanna felt enormous compassion for animals. One day during recess, two boys were threatening to squish a worm. Happening upon the scene, Johanna exclaimed, "Hey! Wait! Worms are life. Killing one worm could change the whole future of a tree! And trees help us live." This complex logic was lost on the eleven-year-old boys, so she swooped down, grabbed the worm, and dashed off. The two boys gave chase, and as Johanna yelled over her shoulder, "I won't let you kill this worm," she carried the worm to safety!

"I am very sensitive to animals hurting or bleeding," Johanna continued. Once, when she was watching an episode of *Animal Planet* with her father, the program's biologists were attempting to net a manta ray suffering from a damaged flipper. In the process of netting the ray, the flipper was torn off. Johanna immediately fainted. With a loud clunk, her head hit the kitchen table. "It affects me deeply when an animal gets hurt, like with a gun. It hurts me on the inside and outside. It hurts me on the inside due to the fact that I feel the animal's pain. That's not right. It's not right to kill things. I'm really sensitive to that kind of stuff." Johanna explained.

Another illustrative example of Johanna's exquisite concern for others' suffering was recounted by her mom: Mother and daughter were in their chiropractor's waiting room. A theatrical toddler, eager to elicit attention with her entertaining antics, pretended to fall on her face. The other adults, appreciating the child's aptitude for acting, broke into laughter. Johanna, on the other hand, was so upset that the toddler might injure herself that she had to adjourn to the car to await her appointment.

Her mother shared that Johanna's language was considerably delayed. In fact, she didn't speak in complete sentences until she was six years old. Also, Johanna routinely had trouble falling asleep at night. Additionally, she experienced recurring headaches. She described the pain as a tight band stretching from ear to ear across her forehead.

Exceptional Features

 Although Johanna had not been formally diagnosed with ASD, she clearly demonstrated many of its hallmark features. Her understanding of social cues seriously undermined her ability to mesh with her peers. This left her feeling sad, and on the fringe during recess. Her language was considerably delayed, and her speech peculiar and odd for an eleven-year-old girl. Johanna's grand passions had changed over the years, but most recently, Bionicles had become her favorite pastime. All of these traits are common to children with ASD.

As homeopaths, we are interested in what distinguishes Johanna from other children with the same diagnosis. We found the intensity of Johanna's sensitivity to others' pain, and her compassion for suffering animals striking. Her ability to empathize with an animal to the point of fainting because she "felt their pain, inside and out," was truly remarkable! There are several medicines for children that empathize strongly with animals' suffering. The one that best fit Johanna was the beautiful yellow water lily, *Nuphar luteum*. Children needing this

medicine exhibit great moral sensibility. They can experience acute pain on witnessing the suffering of animals.
Nuphar luteum is also used to treat the type of headache
Johanna described: a pressing band-like pain across the
forehead.

Gradual but Steady Progress Toward Balance and Happiness

Over the three months after taking her homeopathic
medicine, Johanna's chief concerns improved slowly but
steadily. She reported feeling more patient with the other
kids at school, and felt that she was getting along better
with her classmates. When asked how she felt the homeopathic medicine had helped her, she answered, "It's
helping me make 'half' friends." Johanna's mom noted
she seemed to respond faster when addressed. "Johanna
isn't a responder. We call her or say something to her, and
she normally won't acknowledge us. This is a target area
that has changed. She is more engaged, wanting to be
involved in discussions and activities that don't normally
interest her. Her grades have improved, and she is more
on task."

During this office visit, Johanna expressed a new
concern, "I feel nervous about something, but I don't
know what it is. I feel like I did something wrong," The
child also felt overwhelmed by schoolwork, mainly her
written reports. In spite of this sentiment, Johanna admitted that she was feeling happier in general.

Johanna's homeopathic medicine had moved her in
the right direction. Although the changes were gradual
over the first three months, they were encouraging. We
repeated the *Nuphar*.

Johanna's healing process accelerated further over
the next two months. During our next visit, Johanna
announced that she felt more "laid back" and "cool with

the world." She said she felt more able to "leave things behind" and that everything was going better with other kids. "People don't mind me being around them now," she commented. Johanna added that she had been feeling "more mellow" and not as worried. The feeling of being "nervous about something" had dissolved.

Johanna's mother confirmed the progress. "She's definitely doing a lot better. A tenfold improvement!" She was pleased to report that Johanna had not expressed any suicidal thoughts since starting homeopathic treatment. At this point during Johanna's care, her parents decided to take her off of Ritalin, under the guidance of the prescribing physician.

Johanna's progress continued over the next couple of months. "I haven't had any nightmares since the very first dose," she informed us. "I have made two new friends and it's easy to talk with them. The first time we played was the most fun time I've ever had!" Johanna assured us that she had not been feeling worried or nervous, and was much happier. Her mom agreed with her daughter's observations, but had began to notice how Johanna would interact with adults as if they were equals. "She will debate an adult if she thinks they are wrong," she commented.

During our most recent visit, Johanna informed us that her sleep problems had returned. "I am thinking about how my next day will go," she explained. She had continued to make friends more easily. "The first day of school, I made a new friend. It's as simple as one, two, three! And I think that it is because of my weirdness that they like me!" It warms the heart to see this delightfully compassionate child blossom socially.

However, Johanna did indicate that she had been in a fight with a classmate. "I've been feeling grumpy, I think it's because I'm not getting enough sleep."

Although she was handling most of her other challenges well, because her poor sleep had relapsed, we gave her another dose of *Nuphar*.

Jai: A Proactive Mom Seeks Treatment Prior to Diagnosis

Jai had not yet turned three years old when we started treating him homeopathically. The child displayed many behaviors that foreshadowed a diagnosis of ASD, and his mom, Asha, wanted a drug-free treatment for her son. In addition to suspecting ASD, she feared he was headed for a concurrent diagnosis of ADHD. A vigilant mother, she wanted to be proactive and to get to the root of his problems as quickly as possible. Jai is an example of how, with early treatment, a diagnosis of ASD can be averted.

We began the interview by discussing Asha's pregnancy and Jai's infancy: Jai's birth was difficult—a long labor that didn't progress. He had a posterior position in the birth canal and the obstetrician was unsuccessful in her efforts to turn him. Ultimately, they delivered Jai using forceps. As an infant, Jai seemed overly serious. When others smiled at him and made funny faces, he did not return their greeting. In fact, occasionally the infant frowned and, more often than not, simply looked away disinterestedly.

Cuddling was never high on Jai's priority list. He was content being alone as long as he could do what he wanted. A determined toddler, he asserted his will, regardless of the consequences. "He almost can't control himself." Asha described their interaction as a constant "battle of wills." Insignificant matters, often involving transitions, would set him off. His tantrums, during which Jai threw himself on the floor and screamed for extended periods of time, occurred numerous times each day. He would stiffen his body, stick out his legs, arch his back, and thrash about on the floor. Not a pretty sight. Jai exhibited aggressive behavior toward his younger brother, which worried Asha, "He is very rough with Jayesh", she said. "Jai just pushes him over and doesn't know how to be gentle. He'll attack and not stop."

Me, Myself, and I

Asha described her son as a loner. He appeared to have no desire whatsoever to interact with other children, and tended to gravitate to the periphery to play by himself. Asha elaborated:

> *For example, he doesn't participate in Sunday school 'day care' activities or do what the rest of the group is doing. Jai keeps a straight face during social interactions and doesn't smile much. Sometimes he'll even give an insulting look if people begin talking with him, or he just won't respond. Or he can be rude. If he must have a conversation, his head goes down, and he has a hard time answering their questions.*

With youngsters like Jai, we rely heavily on the parent's keen observation of both behavioral and physical symptoms. A child's sleep pattern, for example, can provide invaluable information—the position he sleeps in, the presence of night terrors, or when he wakes in the night, may be very important to the case. This was true with Jai. He slept warm, and often kicked off the covers during the night. But most striking about Jai's sleep was his copious salivation. He drooled in his sleep, leaving a wet ring of saliva on his pillow in the morning. On rising, he was grumpy and irritable.

Like many kids on the autism continuum, Jai demonstrated an extreme sensitivity to loud noises. Even the sound of the toilet flushing and the bathroom exhaust fan were far too loud for Jai.

A "snarfly" kid, Jai suffered from chronic sinus and lung congestion. Asha was aware of an audible rattle in his chest and throat. When the seasons changed, the stuffiness intensified, and the child blew out excessive amounts of thick, green mucus.

It is understandable that Asha felt concerned about what the future held for the youngster. His poor social interaction skills, aggressiveness, constant and extreme tantrums, and hypersensitivity all pointed to the autism continuum. The combination of her tenacious efforts to identify aggravating dietary influences using the Feingold diet and homeopathy has worked extremely well for Jai.

Thank Goodness for Observant Moms!

Although it can be difficult to take the case of a toddler, Asha's tremendous ability to observe patterns and symptoms in her son enabled us to find the correct homeopathic medicine for him. The child spent time on the periphery rather than being with the group, and would rather look away or frown at someone then make social contact. His unprovoked aggression toward his sibling also stood out.

In addition, Jai exhibited clear physical symptoms. The copious salivation and the subsequent pool of drool in the morning were pronounced. Suspecting a particular homeopathic medicine, we asked, over the phone, that Asha take a look inside Jai's mouth. Sure enough, there were well-defined groove marks along the sides of the boy's tongue. This symptom helped to confirm our choice of the homeopathic medicine.

Exceptional Features

 We prescribed for Jai homeopathic *Mercurius* (mercury), a medicine frequently used for introverted children who do not make social contact easily. (Although mercury can be toxic in its crude form, it is completely safe when prepared homeopathically.) These youngsters sometimes view others as enemies, and, judging from how Jai responded to friendly social cues, and his unprovoked attacks on his brother, we wondered if this might be his perception of the world around him. We were not able to explore this hypothesis in depth with Jai due to his limited conversational abilities. Children needing *Mercurius* can be hesitant, discontented, and averse to transition. They dislike criticism and contradiction, and can be quick to respond with anger or aggression.

On a physical level, Jai's copious nocturnal salivation and his indented tongue are hallmarks of *Mercurius*, as is the excessive thick, green nasal discharge. Finally, children needing *Mercurius* are prone to becoming easily overheated at night, and may kick off their covers, just like Jai.

Happiness is a Warm Hello

Jai's response to his homeopathic medicine was gradual, but profound. Sometimes we see changes on the physical level before the behaviors are affected. This was the case with Jai. During the first six-week follow-up appointment, Jai's mom noted that his sinus problems were completely gone. She also observed that the salivation at night had decreased considerably, and that his snoring had stopped. His socializing was a bit better.

After three months, Asha reported as follows. "He is fidgety," she told us, "but hasn't been having as many tantrums." At the four-month point, she added that he was better able to sit still and was less irritable. The boy was now sleeping soundly through the night, and had stopped twirling his hair compulsively, which had not been mentioned initially. Another positive change was the absence of wetting himself during the day, also skipped over in the original case. This is an example of how focused many parents are, during the first appointment, on the ASD symptoms rather than the physical complaints. It also points out how the correct homeopathic medicine can address these symptoms even if the parents forget to mention them.

At his five-month consultation, Asha shared, "He's still shy with a roomful of people, but is socializing better in general. He is acting more friendly towards people. In fact, if someone approaches him, he'll throw up his hands and exclaim 'Hey!' He smiles more, tells me he feels happy, and just seems happier!" Jai's aggressive overtures towards his brother had diminished markedly. This is music to the ears of a homeopath, especially in Jai's case! We knew we were on the right track with the *Mercurius*.

A New Symptom Picture Calls for a New Medicine

Asha was very pleased with the steady strides Jai had made toward health, yet we both agreed that he had reached a plateau. He was requiring a re-dose every three weeks, and we felt we could find a medicine that had a more sustained effect. Additionally, after the recent increase in the potency of *Mercurius*, he began to experience nosebleeds. We identified this as a proving symptom rather than a natural symptom of Jai's. Proving symptoms are "add-on" symptoms that immediately go away when the medicine is discontinued. This was the case with Jai; his nosebleeds stopped when we switched medicines, and have not returned since.

At this point, we stepped back to take a new look at the case, identify what symptoms had persisted, and what symptoms were new. Asha described Jai's cross demeanor and irritability. At times, he could not stand being looked at, and would scream, "Don't look at me! Don't talk to me!" Asha described how Jai's body would stiffen during an outburst, his arms and legs sticking out. Asha was unable to console Jai during these tantrums. On a physical level, Jai had been grinding his teeth at night, and was waking up in the morning very hungry.

These symptoms provided a clear indication for a medicine called *Cina* (wormseed). Children needing *Cina* can be very cross and are inconsolable during tantrums. They hate being looked at or touched, and will stiffen with anger when either happens. Additionally, Jai's teeth grinding and extreme hunger provided good physical confirmation that Jai needed a dose of *Cina*.

Asha was very pleased with the changes she observed in Jai after the *Cina*. "He seems happier, he's interacting with people and has been more communicative." Asha noted that Jai had been eating out at restaurants, and did fine with it, including fried foods. In fact, he ate at a Chinese restaurant (a Feingold Diet no-no) without a problem. Also, Asha mentioned that Jai's bowel function had improved considerably.

We've treated Jai for nearly two years, and though he still has his occasional off-days, Asha has estimated his overall improvement to be "at least 90% better, almost normal! A lot of things are clicking for him!"

7

Preoccupied and Persistent
Trains, Planes, and Bionicles

Many an ASD child's apparently limitless grasp of one particular subject causes jaws to drop in amazement. How curious it is that a five-year-old can recite, in a flatly encyclopedic manner, more than you might ever care to know about every train engine that was ever built from 1817 to the present. Other ASD kids may engage you in seemingly never-ending conversations about light switch plates, or dinosaur eggs, or ceiling fans. It is downright puzzling to most NT adults that anyone could develop such a persistent interest in such a specialized subject, much less want to read, talk, and focus on that one subject day and night.

If your child were merely silently fixated on his grand passion, it might be manageable. But when he insists on relentlessly instructing and interrogating everyone around him about his passion, the situation can pretty quickly seem out of hand. At first, a parent may find the breadth of the child's knowledge base fascinating. But, hour after hour, day after day of incessant badgering about this sole topic, to the exclusion of everything else, can get old fast. Of course, you want to foster your child's interests any way you can, but seeing his world narrow so microscopically can be disconcerting. It is also painful to witness your child's futile attempts to engage other children, family friends, or the stranger he happens to meet in the grocery line, with the same outpouring of unsolicited information about plumbing connections, tea bags, or drill bit manufacturers.

Such kids are often brilliant, yet they may be clueless as to how their constant verbal barrage or persistent activity affect those around them. You might wonder how it would be if you could only harness and direct this remarkable talent for gathering information in a way that benefited, rather than isolated him. Such a channeled direction might be available later in life for many ASD adults, as noted autistic writer Temple Grandin found with innovative work designing more humane cattle chutes.

Homeopathy can help the ASD child temper these passions in a positive way, so that they no longer stand in the way of relating to others. Most people with ASD— both children and adults—will always have some kind of strong, focused interest. This can be part of their strengths (where would Edison or Einstein have been without that driving interest?). But homeopathic treatment can help ASD kids draw the line between a fascination that informs and a persistent behavior (perseveration) that interferes with other aspects of their lives.

Tito: Monsters, Blood, and Nothing Else

Tito, seven years old and diagnosed with AS and OCD, lived several thousand miles away, so the appointments were conducted by phone. Though we never laid eyes on Tito in person, he came alive to us, as he surely will to you.

"Friendly, charming, and likeable" were the words Tito's mom, Anna, first used to describe him to us seven years ago. This boy was so sensitive that "you could break his heart in two seconds." Like when he tried to make friends and couldn't. He nearly collapsed if told he did something wrong. The most curious feature of Tito's case was his fascination, to the point of obsession, with blood and gore. His mother, a gentle soul who was frankly embarrassed by the violent nature of her son's impassioned focus of interest, described it in vivid detail:

> *The monster thing—that's him. Tito is forever talking about monsters. The blood gushing out. How he cut somebody's throat. My son first got into monster storybooks when he was two. I thought it was funny at the beginning. When he started school at three and a half, he was traumatized. The kids bullied him for a year. He got beaten up every single day. Tito was accident-prone anyway. When another child kicked him in the mouth, he lost his two front teeth.*

Tito used scary stories to defend himself and became known as the school storyteller. His tales were so scary that the school complained about other youngsters being unable to sleep because his stories were so frightening. "Tito comes by it naturally", his mother explained. "My husband is a writer, and Tito inherited his father's creativity. Either someone would die in his stories or the tales would have no ending at all. Like this: 'It was dark. A boy was walking through the forest. He found an alien's house. The alien had lots of hands. A big hand came reaching out. The alien spit poison. The boy died.' They even scare me, and I'm his mom."

Diagnosed initially with obsessive-compulsive disorder, then with bipolar disorder, his final diagnosis was AS. Fascinated with the notion of drinking blood, Tito picked at his arms until they bled. He loved to recount tales involving cutting, carving, or Dracula. At the age of two, Anna bought him a vampire costume for Halloween. Tito refused to wear anything else for months. Elaborating to no end on how blood tasted and how blood came out of this or that person's throat, Tito would gently grab Anna's neck at the supermarket to act out his tales. The boy could be in the car driving to the store with his mom when he would launch into one of his gruesome stories, without even noticing when she got out of the car to fill the gas tank. Upon her return, the youngster had continued his narration without interruption, as if she had not even left. If his stories weren't about blood, they focused on fights and violence. Tito explained to his mom that he often had a Goosebumps movie going on inside his head. Thanks to a nearly photographic memory, learning a poem took Tito a matter of seconds, but it didn't capture his attention unless it was scary.

A Creative Escape from Bullying
Ironically, Tito was anything but aggressive. A blue belt in karate, he would not even consider hurting another child. Tito could count only one friend at school. From the time he entered preschool, the other kids either ignored or harassed the child. The psychologist described him as withdrawn and a loner. Tito chattered incessantly. Lost in his world of bloody fantasy, he would exclaim, "I'm gonna cut your neck and drink your blood." Though charming with adults, conversation quickly broke down whenever Tito tried to talk to peers, and he found himself alone on the playground, in the classroom, or in the lunchroom. The cool kids simply told Tito to get lost. Despite his bloody bravado, the boy was quite sensitive and the callous treatment severely injured his tender feelings.

Verbally precocious, though only seven years old, Tito possessed the language skills of a tenth grader. Nevertheless, he attended a school for learning-disabled children. Also diagnosed as dyslexic, Tito's handwriting was disorganized, and many of his letters were written backwards. When asked to draw a human figure, all the limbs radiated from the head of whomever he depicted.

Phobic of germs, Tito scrambled out of the room if he heard anyone cough. A frequent hand washer and compulsive teeth brusher, the child could not tolerate anyone touching his food. "Germs" was almost as common a word in his vocabulary as "blood." Tito was terrified of being buried alive or grabbed in a dark cave. The mere sight of a dog would send him running to hide. Whenever Tito left the house with his mom, he feared losing her. He also awakened regularly between two and four in the morning to look for her. Upon finding her, Tito insisted that she tell him over and over that she loved him. Tito was afraid of being hit by another child whenever he left the house. Other fears included sharks, man-o-wars, and ants. Every night, Tito escaped to the comfort and security of his parents' bed. He talked of special friends who lived in an imaginary attic and came down whenever he needed their help.

A chilly, wiry child, Tito suffered from asthma, chronic ear infections, and recurrent bronchitis. He had been on Amoxicillin frequently from age two to four. Headaches were his current chief complaint, particularly when he needed to make choices, even simple ones like whether he wanted a red cup or a white one. Bedwetting had continued until age six and a half.

Tito's mother recounted that she had taken Xanax during the first two months of her pregnancy, and had been convinced that the baby would suffer brain damage as a result. Labor went fine until the birthing team lost his heartbeat, and prepped his mom for an emergency C-section, at which time she quickly gave birth to Tito vaginally.

Slow to develop, Tito rarely cried, and was unusually passive from infancy to the present. At one year of age, the pediatrician informed Anna that her son possessed the fine motor skills of a three-month-old. With regard to gross motor skills, however, Tito was unable to grab even a raisin, and his walking was delayed until fifteen months.

Exceptional Features

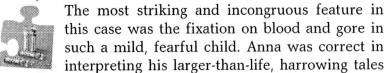

The most striking and incongruous feature in this case was the fixation on blood and gore in such a mild, fearful child. Anna was correct in interpreting his larger-than-life, harrowing tales as a compensation for his own timidity and terror. In the homeopathic literature, Tito's fascination is expressed as "excitement at hearing horrible things."

The homeopathic medicine *China* (Peruvian bark) fits this characteristic, and is indicated for individuals who feel harassed and persecuted, which was certainly true of Tito. The medicine is also indicated for people who experience a fear of dogs and have dreams and impulses regarding knives. *China* was the very first substance proved by Dr. Samuel Hahnemann, the founder of homeopathy. There is a wealth of information concerning this medicine. A member of the *Rubiaceae* family, the members of this group are useful medicines for people who are over-stimulated mentally, their minds overflowing with creative ideas, daydreams, and plans. Children who are highly sensitive to their environments often need a homeopathic medicine derived from a plant, rather than an animal or mineral. As with most of the children we treat, we prescribed a single dose of the medicine to be taken once.

A Rapid Response

Although our first follow-ups are typically six weeks after the initial appointment, Anna did not schedule a follow-up call until nearly three months later. Tito had an excellent response to the *China* for two months, then relapsed after receiving an injection of antibiotics for a strep throat. Immediately after taking the *China*, he had become briefly hyperactive, smashing two of his toys and, curiously, put his bicycle in his parents' bed. Then, within days, "The monster thing disappeared completely," according to his mother. Before, when his little sister asked Tito to read her a story, it had always been exclusively monster stories and nothing else. Now he read Dr. Seuss to her instead. The boy began reading more easily than ever before and, "like magic, began to be aware of what was around him."

On the sixth day after taking the *China*, he grabbed a piece of paper and hastily wrote out three pages of karate techniques. Tito's reading improved remarkably. His teacher asked him to read one book and, instead, he read ten. Both mom and dad described the change in their son as "incredible." Following the antibiotics, Tito was pretty much back to how he had been before taking the *China*, though his reading remained excellent.

Conventional drug treatment, such as antibiotics, can sometimes interfere with homeopathic treatment. In his case, the antibiotics did trigger a relapse, so the *China* was administered once more.

This time Tito did not experience an aggravation. He returned to talking some about monsters, but not to the same extent as before, and there was no mention whatsoever of blood. The child's reading skills improved "like day and night" so that his teacher commented that she saw no evidence of a learning disability. Tito was even nominated for an all-school award. His handwriting became legible. Noticeably less anxious, he stopped picking at his arm. Tito dreamed of slashing a four-armed monster with an axe. The obsession with monsters and blood was now being acted out subconsciously in his dreams, rather than in his waking state.

From "Prospective Serial Killer" to Gifted Child

We repeated the *China* again eight months after the original dose because some of Tito's original symptoms had returned, but to a much lesser degree. By this time the youngster was attending public school in a mainstream classroom with gifted children and was considered one of the best students. His expressive language was much better, and he now had several friends.

Tito's mom recalled, at this time, that a prominent psychologist in their area had previously warned her that Tito had the profile of a serial killer. He had based this assessment on the fixation with slashing and bloodletting. By this time all Tito's diagnoses had changed. The only label that fit him now was that of a gifted child.

We treated Tito over the course of two years. His conversational skills progressed steadily. His storytelling evolved into a wonderful talent for writing. Even when the characters were monsters, which happened occasionally, there was no blood. They became "just a small part of his life." The youngster developed a love of basketball and dreamed of becoming either a "great basketball player or an actor." Or, he added, "if those two careers don't work out, a writer."

Jared: Mismatched Ability and Performance

Jared, a bright, lovable, carrot-topped, seven-year-old youngster with impressive artistic talent, came for treatment for his attention problems, food sensitivities, and perfectionism. Jared daydreamed in school, and had trouble focusing and staying on task. On the playground, he tended to become giddy.

The child's teachers marveled that, in all their years of teaching, they had never seen another child like him. His verbal IQ tested at 122, despite feedback from the school psychologist that he was barely paying attention during the testing. As a result, Jared's performance IQ tested at only 91. These IQ scores are similar to other children with AS—in that ability and performance are mismatched. Although Jared had not been formally diagnosed with AS, a number of features of his case, including special interests, limited social skills, and obsessive tendencies point strongly to such a diagnosis.

Whenever Jared made a mistake he would apologize for being a failure. Highly self-critical, he believed that his mistakes were a source of deep disappointment to his parents. If he received all outstanding grades except for one, he became very upset that his report card was less than perfect. Jared was an anxious child, and was fearful of trying anything new. The youngster was also afraid of burglars, water, bees and wasps, mosquito eaters, and spiders, especially poisonous ones.

He Drew Up to Fifty Pictures a Day

Jared's mom described him as an exceptionally creative boy, a talented artist who loved to draw. Because Jared was prone to fixate on certain interests for periods of time, his drawings focused one month on police cars, the next on dinosaurs or wild cats. His detailed, three-dimensional images of dinosaurs and big cats, complete with teeth and claws, were quite impressive. Astoundingly, Jared created up to fifty pictures a day. His aspiration was to become a famous artist. Even with his talent, however, the boy had refused to draw at school until he got a

Magna-Doodle, a magnetic drawing board that allowed him to erase his mistakes easily. Sensitive to artificial colors and flavors and salicylate-containing foods, Jared had benefited from adhering to the Feingold Diet, which excludes food additives, preservatives, and dyes. Offending foods caused him to become very hyperactive and to act like a tiger, growling, snarling, and pounding his fist against his hand or head. Jared exhibited limited social skills, and found it difficult to recognize social cues. As a result, he had only one good friend, who himself suffered from ADD. An affectionate child, Jared would crawl into his mother's lap and tell her sweetly that he loved her. In fact, he hugged others to the point of getting into trouble. Hearing-impaired as a result of chronic ear infections early in his life, the boy wore hearing aids in class.

Jared was wise beyond his years. He was a virtual encyclopedia of information and frequently began his sentences with "Did you know that...?" As intelligent and artistic as Jared was, he was not physically adept. Hesitant to attempt new physical activities for fear of getting hurt, Jared rode his scooter around the neighborhood, but lacked the courage to learn to ride a bicycle.

Jared had a nervous habit of nail biting, and chewed his nails down to the quick, even to the point of bleeding. He occasionally wet the bed, which embarrassed him. Also remarkable were his numerous moles, and a prominent *café-au-lait*-colored birthmark on his chest. Jared's mom described a strong history of cancer on both sides of Jared's family, including cancers of the breast, lung, colon, stomach and throat.

Lions, Tigers, and T-Rexes
When we interviewed Jared alone, he shared how much he enjoyed drawing, reading, and writing. Fascinated by

lions, tigers, and dinosaurs, Jared elaborated, "I think of all the dinosaurs I can imagine. I hold them still, in a pause way, and sketch everything. It turns out to be the right thing. When I find a plastic dinosaur, I think of how it could fight. The stegosaurus swings his tail at the allosaur, but the allosaur eats the stegosaurus. The allosaur goes 'R-a-a-a-h!'"

Jared described in detail how he had created his own alien out of animal parts from a T-Rex, a cheetah, an eagle and a stegosaurus. He explained he was working on a movie called *Jurassic Park: The Allosaur Returns*. The screenplay's theme was quite similar to other installments in the series, in which the humans try to shoot the dinosaur, who turns on them, and eats them all. We were not surprised to learn that Jared also had scary dreams of dinosaurs, "There's excitement in them!" he exclaimed. When asked if he would like to travel anywhere, Jared responded, "Sure. Six Flags and Jurassic Park!" Jared continued:

> *Sometimes I draw evil things, like evil men and women. Or I draw snakes as big as two men, or lizards as small as ants. If I make a mistake in my drawings, I kind of feel bad. I don't like it. Anger comes to my mind and I get upset or go 'g-r-r-r'. If I get in trouble, I feel, 'Oh, no!' I could get suspended from school!*

Special Features

Jared has needed only one homeopathic medicine over the course of the past two years: *Carcinosin* (a nosode). A child needing *Carcinosin* may come from a family in which the expectations are very high—so high that the youngster may feel he has to push himself beyond his capacity in order to fulfill them. The child becomes sensitive to any situation that might suggest he is less than perfect. The mere suggestion that he had made a mistake confirmed his belief that he was a failure. Upset if he did anything at all that might disappoint his parents or teacher, any and all situations, such as drawing in school prior to acquiring his Magna-Doodle, held the potential for mistakes.

Those needing this medicine are typically creative, artistically talented, bright, and intense. They may excel in the arts, including music, drama, dance, and art. Jared had a great imagination, expressed vividly and visually in his detailed animal drawings, as well as his ideas for dinosaur movies. We find these kids to be affectionate, sympathetic, and kind, like Jared. He also loved to travel, another typical symptom of children needing this medicine. Another classic feature of those needing this medicine is moles, birthmarks, and *café-au-lait* spots or *latte*-colored skin.

The Body Heals Itself After the Correct Medicine

Six weeks later, Jared's mother reported that his bedwetting had stopped for the first fourteen days, then returned after he became upset with himself. After another ten days, Jared was noticeable calmer and easier on himself, able to relax for the first time in months, and more loving than ever. The nail biting now occurred only during moments of overexcitement. A transient, red rash appeared under his armpits, along with few bumps under his nose and in the vicinity of his *café-au-lait* birthmark. Such skin eruptions soon after taking a homeopathic medicine are usually a good indicator that the medicine is the correct one.

At his third visit, Jared's mother related her surprise that the holes that had remained in his eardrums following the surgical insertion of ear tubes (a treatment for chronic ear infections) had repaired themselves, resulting in slightly improved hearing. The boy was steadily able to handle disappointments without self-reproach, and better able to reason out situations that were not going his way. Far less thin-skinned when it came to criticism, Jared did a show-and-tell in our office of several free-hand illustrations of dinosaurs and big cats. The drawings were excellent, well beyond his years in detail and artistic ability.

At the next visit we gave Jared a higher dose of *Carcinosin* because the improvements, though significant, had reached a plateau. His attentiveness in the classroom had wavered, which caused him frustration. "I get mad at myself for not being perfect," he lamented. Jared shared with us some dreams of dinosaurs and golden treasures. Soon after taking the medicine, the skin eruptions again appeared, then quickly disappeared, on various areas of his body. Focus was definitely better, allowing Jared to complete an advanced science fair project that would not previously have been possible for him. Now he could laugh about not being perfect, and confided, "I'm not getting angry if I make a mistake. I don't think I have to get everything perfect anymore."

We have treated Jared over the past two and a half years, and he has needed a dose of *Carcinosin* every two to three months. His food sensitivities to additives, preservatives, and salicylates have decreased markedly. The bedwetting and nail biting have not returned. The boy suffered one sudden and dramatic relapse after he was accused of not turning in his homework. He again felt a sense of worthlessness, as he had prior to homeopathic treatment. This self-deprecation turned around immediately after another dose of *Carcinosin*. Jared's grades are high and, finishing fourth grade, he reads at a seventh-grade level. The last time we saw Jared, he summed it up quite nicely. "I feel more relaxed and peaceful. I'm happier with where I am. I'm not bothered by anything anymore."

Drew: Weird Faces and Goofy Behavior

Diagnosed at a pediatric hospital with autism at the age of four, and later with ADHD, Drew's problems had eluded his parents because he was able to blend in so well. A very passive infant, it wasn't until a medical profession pointed out what she called the "soft signs" of autism that it dawned on them that something was amiss. Drew talked when he was moved to do so. Otherwise, he rarely uttered a word. The youngster was placed in a kindergarten class for developmentally delayed children. The child had two other siblings, the oldest of whom has since been diagnosed with AS. Shortly before we first saw Drew, his diagnosis was changed from autism to AS.

Maggie, Drew's mom, shared with us openly:

My goal was healing and recovery. The diagnosis of autism is not something I shared with his peers. I was very reluctant to have Drew assessed cognitively, because if he weren't typical, I didn't think I could bear having a second child who had developmental and learning problems. Drew's testing came back as superior cognitively in all areas. In fact, though he was only in the third grade, he was reading at a ninth-grade level. Drew's grades were mostly As and some Bs. He has always been quite serious academically. I'm a special-ed teacher myself, so I'm aware of the delineations. Drew tests one level below gifted. My hopes are that he can become a scientist or an engineer. He performs fine in a structured setting.

Drew has been on Concerta for the past two years for ADHD. We stopped giving it to him because it kept him up at night. He also takes a morning dose of Ritalin. Without the stimulants, Drew acts like he has Tourette's. He sticks out his tongue, cocks his head, and makes faces. The Concerta kind of reined him in. But Drew just isn't a child that parents feel like inviting over to play with their kids. The parents don't like him because he's so different. 'Goofy' is the word they usually use. Drew decided yesterday it would be funny to pretend to spray the congregation with artillery fire while singing a song and making faces at the people. He loses the fact that there are a hundred people looking at him.

Maggie offered a classic example of Drew's behavior. The family had gone to the movies the previous Friday evening. Drew spotted a girl that he knew and immediately put his head right next to hers while making babyish facial expressions and "preverbal *gee, gaw, goo* sounds." He found the incident entertaining, and was oblivious to the girl's discomfort.

Drew did not speak by the age of four, prompting his parents to enroll him in an extensive speech therapy program. When the youngster started kindergarten, he showed no interest in connecting with his classmates. Now he did, but they had no desire to be around *him*. In fact, they made fun of Drew, smashed his projects, and rarely invited him to their birthday parties. The other kids pushed Drew while they were in line to get fitted for ice skates and kicked him when the teacher wasn't looking. Drew responded by withdrawing, "making weird faces," and talking to himself. Like many other children with ASD, Drew was clumsy, fell easily and often, and hated sports, except for ice skating.

He Reads the Encyclopedia for Fun

Whenever Drew read a book, he first carefully pored over the index to determine exactly what interested him. He spent a good three to four hours a day perusing the encyclopedia and devouring facts about dinosaurs, Greek myths, and whatever other subject caught his fancy at the moment. In conversation with his parents, he politely informed or corrected them. Like providing the historical and biographical information regarding Bacchus and Filomena. If a topic came up that no one knew the answer to, you could be sure that Drew would thoroughly research the question, then come back and supply the correct data. His parents were quite pleased with his intellectual prowess, though he would sometimes lecture them in a rather condescending manner. Adults generally found Drew to be fascinating and highly instructive. Though some parents talked to or about him as if he were mentally retarded, his pedantic nature only served to further alienate his classmates, who already considered him strange. It is not surprising that, academically Drew "blew the other kids out of the water."

Taking Drew out in public presented a challenge for his parents.

You're always afraid of what he's going to do. Once he hit another child with a shovel at a Cub Scout meeting. Another time his brother pulled down Drew's pants while they were on the playground during recess and the youngster hadn't a clue that he should pull them back up. Then there was pajama day at school when Drew forgot to wear his underwear underneath his pajamas. His dad's stomach is

in knots when he takes him to a scout meeting
because he never knows what to expect.
We live in a rather snotty neighborhood and pre-
fer to say nothing about our son having autism. We
walk on eggshells because everyone else on our
block who has been different has ended up moving
away.

Drew had a fascination with guns, and was beginning to exhibit aggressive tendencies. Once when Maggie
told him she didn't have enough change for a doughnut,
he raised his arm to strike her. Drew had recently kicked
in the door of his Sunday school classroom. He had also
become increasingly reactive towards a bully who was
habitually victimizing him at school.

Dreams of Explosions, Spaceships, Murders, and Fires
What first impressed us were Drew's beautiful facial features, and his habit of fidgeting restlessly throughout the
interview. The child told us that he had a hard time going
to sleep at night because of his fear of nightmares. And
that his brother "was egging him on to act goofy and to
make stupid faces and sounds." He proceeded, spontaneously, to launch into a detailed description of his vivid
dreams. They often involved a spaceship or some other
vehicle or object blowing up or catching fire. Somehow
the driver or pilot remained unharmed, despite extraordinary flight paths directly through mountains or pyra-
mids. Some of his dreams made references to "growling,
showing your claws, biting, squeezing, beating out the
stuffing and intestines, and being captured." These powerful dreams had such an impact on Drew that he
thought them to be real, even after waking up. This type
of dream had special significance in light of the homeopathic medicine we ended up prescribing for Drew. Over

and over he referred to being hunted down, and of someone or something trying to eat him or do something bad
to him. Drew could have easily spent an hour or more
expounding elaborately on his dreams. When the subject
turned to school, Drew painted a rosy picture. He denied
being bullied by others and could not remember a time
during recess when the other children mistreated him.
The youngster even insisted that he had plenty of friends,
which was clearly not the case. We surmised that it was
just too embarrassing for him to tell us the painful truth
about his social ostracism. Drew also told us that he was
very fond of cats.

Exceptional Features

Drew was remarkably bright, articulate, and
imaginative, and he exhibited the typical AS
pedantic, professorial tendency. His habits of
putting himself right in the faces of his peers,
and of making odd grimaces, gestures, and noises was not
at all unusual among the ASD population. Although
Drew was the only child we have met so far to devour the
encyclopedia for several hours at a time, his passion for
knowledge, though extreme, was not something new to
our ears. What seemed most curious were the recurrent,
vivid, violent dreams. They were so intense that he was
afraid to go to sleep at night.

The first medicine that we prescribed was
Stramonium (thorn apple), one of the most common
homeopathic medicines for intense, fearful, violent children. The fears of a child needing this medicine often
include wild animals, the dark, and water. Though there
was a definite benefit from the medicine, we were not
completely satisfied and gave three other medicines a
trial before settling on the final one, which has helped

Drew the most dramatically over the past nine months. We will first describe the child's positive response to *Stramonium* before illustrating the benefit he derived from his most recent prescription.

Better Speech and Eye Contact, Then a Relapse

Within an hour of taking *Stramonium*, Drew's speech was noticeably different. (It usually takes days to weeks before the effects of homeopathy are obvious, but some patients report a definite shift within minutes or hours.) That evening his eye contact improved. Drew blushed for the first time in his life. His behavior and conversation was more appropriate, and his tendency to fixate dramatically lessened. In place of the childish jokes he had told before, now he talked to his mother in a much more mature fashion. Drew told his mom that he was very happy she had taken him for homeopathic treatment. The all-around improvement lasted for a little over a month. Maggie noticed a regression shortly after he drank some of his dad's coffee. (It is common knowledge among homeopaths that, in some patients, coffee can interrupt the positive effect of a homeopathic medicine.) Maggie reported after six weeks,

You would not believe what we've seen. It has been so thrilling. His father was totally amazed, too. He was a different Drew. The kids who shunned him are now playing basketball with him. Right after taking the medicine, he was more aggressive for a day or two. Then, there was this wonderful period for a month. The kid who was always inside that we never saw came out. His last report card showed improvement in twenty different areas. He got seventeen As. Before drinking the coffee, he was actually hanging out with the other kids at church.

The Tourette symptoms were gone. Now they've begun again. He is again saying repetitive, goofy things. In the past week he's crawling around on the floor howling, and he chased a neighbor boy with a bat. The disconnectedness with others is back and his speech is more choppy again. The babyish quality is back.

We asked Drew how he had felt since the homeopathic treatment. He replied that he felt more in control instead of being a "goofball and out of whack." He acknowledged that he was able to play with more kids and that his self-esteem was better.

The *Stramonium* was repeated. Over the following nine months, Drew continued to progress, but not to the extent that we knew was possible. The child continued to have disturbing, violent dreams, including more dreams of being hunted down, which prevented him from going to sleep easily. We tried three other medicines without a significant further improvement.

The Puzzle Pieces Come Together

By mid-December, 2003, Drew was having some good days and some bad days at school. The original dramatic improvements had lasted only partially. Although much about Drew was undeniably better than before beginning homeopathy, we were not satisfied. He told us about his urges to throw cups at people's heads, steal food, and "concoct huge messes."

The habit of stealing food caught our attention. We also explored in depth the feeling of being chased. Drew explained that he didn't like using up all of his muscles and fuel. It felt to him as if there were a little, magnetic tracking device that allowed others to get him. He used, as he had before, a number of animal images, which made us wonder if he might, in fact, need a homeopathic medicine made from an animal source. This was confirmed when he repeated words such as *the pursuer, sneak up on you, stalk, hide,* and *pounce.* When we explored this subject line further, Drew spoke clearly of someone getting him while his back was turned, of his being surrounded, grabbed, and stealthily overpowered. "They sneak up and kill you. You're hunched down, below eye level. Then everybody shoots. You jump up on the person and attack him. You claw him. Like my cat." At this point Drew made a ferocious big-cat-like gesture. "Then they kill you." Drew provided steadily more clues to identify the animal that he was describing—big claws, sharp teeth, vicious, and a pitch-black color, in order to be camouflaged in the dark.

It was clear that he was using the same words again and again, and that the images had come to life. We prescribed homeopathic *Panther.* (Rest assured that homeopathic mammal medicines are made from a drop of blood or milk so that no harm is done to the animal providing the sample.)

That was nine months ago and Drew has continued to respond dramatically. Within two months of the original dose, Drew was getting along much better with his peers—no fighting, kicking, or shoving. He shared that there just wasn't much that annoyed him anymore because his tolerance was better. The chasing theme in the child's dreams had been replaced by the occasional UFO or spaceship. Dads are generally harder sells than moms when it comes to acknowledging improvement in their kids, but Drew's dad affirmed that his son was much more easy-going since the *Panther.* His attentiveness was significantly improved. He had even invited his "mortal enemy" to his house to play a few weeks earlier, and they got along famously. Maggie shared that Drew seemed much more peaceful and happy. His behavior was noticeably more flexible when things didn't go according to his plan.

Drew needed one more dose of the *Panther* six months after the first dose when some of his symptoms began to return. That dose set him back on course. Since that time, the youngster is much more able to assess relationships with others and to sort out friendships for himself. Happier, more interactive, and just plain fun to be around, Drew's lost the goofy, alienating behaviors he once displayed. He was "just one of the guys" at vacation Bible school and fit right in at a church camp-out. He has become much more interested in going out and being with people. He actually asks to accompany Maggie when she goes out to do errands. Drew is much more willing to experiment with different foods, and has learned to keep his mouth closed when he eats. Although his eye contact still has room for improvement and Maggie describes his speech as "still jagged, not linear", the youngster has made tremendous strides with homeopathic treatment.

8

Odd and Obsessive
Hand Washing, Twirling, and Counting

Children with ASD sometimes attempt to manage an unpredictable, disorderly world by calming themselves with repetitive and obsessive activities such as hand flapping, twirling, and counting. Parents can often gauge their child's stress level by how much time she spends engaged in her "self-stimming," slang for self-stimulation. Unfortunately, such mannerisms and behaviors are perceived as unusual and unacceptable by other children. Even parents are pushed to the limit of their patience when the flapping and twirling become so repetitive as to become a focal point of the day.

Obsessive Compulsive Disorder (OCD), though different from self-stimming, can involve repetitive or ritualistic behaviors such as compulsive hand washing. Like self-stimming, they can become an embarassment and a cause for alienation in an already different child.

The cases in this chapter are examples of how homeopathy can help reduce these tendencies. With homeopathic treatment, we typically find that the child is more easily able to blend in with peers and the public, and feels more relaxed and comfortable. Ultimately, the stress level of both parents and child is diminished.

Chris: Barreling Into His Classmates at Eighty Miles an Hour

Chris, now six years old, had been helped considerably by his previous homeopath, who felt she had done as much as she could and referred him to us. At three days of age, Chris had spiked a 100-degree fever, and was taken back to the hospital, where a spinal tap and CT scan were found to be normal. Chris's doting mom, Jenny, breastfed her son until he was five months, but each feeding was an ordeal. The infant nursed five minutes, screamed for half an hour, then suckled again. As an infant, he slept only 45 minutes at a time. Night terrors started at one year and "extended tantrums" at eighteen months. Chris was known to shriek for up to two and a half hours straight in the middle of the night in addition to his daytime meltdowns. His parents, who described their little darling as "mad as heck with the universe" were exhausted. As a toddler, Chris was just plain angry. All of his baby pictures show him grimacing.

Chris uttered his first sentence at nine or ten months. In contrast, physical milestones such as walking, graduating from a high chair, and getting rid of his bicycle training wheels were difficult. Jenny explained, "Christopher was born thirty-five years old. He won't do a thing until he's darned ready."

Social interactions were tough from the start. Chris showed little respect for other children's boundaries, invading their space by hugging, touching, grabbing, and shoving. Chris liked to always run the show, which drove would-be friends away in frustration. Though he genuinely wanted playmates, Chris had no understanding of the normal give and take required to maintain friendships. When lucky enough to have a buddy, Chris would slug any other child who sat next to his friend. On the playground, Chris was overly enthusiastic, barreling into his classmates at eighty miles an hour.

When social situations turned sour, Chris sulked, grimaced, hit, shrugged, and yelled. "They're being mean to me" or "They don't like me. I don't have any friends. Nobody wants to play with me." Teachers and caregivers loved Chris, but were exasperated by him. His thinking process was way beyond his years, yet his social skills were considerably delayed. Teacher comments typically indicated that Chris had "huge potential, wanted to be good, and tried hard."

Pterodactyls in the Bedroom and Sharks in the Bathroom

An inveterate worrier, Chris needed continual reassurance from his mother that pterodactyls and alligators would not climb up into his room and get him. Watching TV further fueled Chris' fears and obsessions. Little did his kindergarten teacher realize that her teaching unit on germs would leave the child germ-phobic. His exaggerated concern led to ritual hand washing thirty to fifty times a day. Touching his underpants, even the elastic, was intolerable. If Chris touched something with his right hand, he needed to touch it with his left hand also. The same ritual applied to climbing his bunk bed ladder—first the right toe, then the left, and so on. Chris riddled his weary mom with a seemingly endless barrage of questions, such as why other kids didn't like him and whether sharks would come into the bathroom to eat him.

Chris' father, Jim, pointed out that he and his son shared much in common. Neither liked crowds. Both were resistant to ideas the first time they heard them. Neither father nor son "suffered fools," and were quite sure that *they* knew more than anyone else did. Chris' paternal grandfather checked locks obsessively each night before retiring and would drive back home if he thought he had left a door unlocked. Jim had exhibited ritualized touching and hand washing earlier in his life, and still checked every door and window in the house at bedtime. Afraid of the dark well into his twenties, Jim was also frightened by monsters, heights, the unknown, and situations he couldn't control. Chris, similarly, was reluctant to try anything the least bit dangerous, refusing to even watch the scary parts of Disney movies. Only in the past year would he begin to venture forth on a jungle gym.

Chris reacted to ingesting corn products by developing bright red cheeks, uncontrollably spinning "like a dervish," and racing up and down the hallways. Eliminating corn-containing foods for a year helped, but with two high-energy boys only two years apart, maintaining a restrictive diet became too cumbersome for the family. In addition to being sensitive to a number of foods, Chris was easily overstimulated by noises, light, rough clothing, and crowds. The boy was physically sensitive as well: at age four and a half, Chris suffered from shingles, for which he was given a one-week course of AZT, a well-known AIDS medication.

Exceptional Features

Chris had many characteristics of AS, including speech delay, difficulties with social interactions, a susceptibility to overstimulation, persistent behavior, and a lack of appreciation of personal boundaries. At his first appointment, we broached the possibility of AS. Chris' mom, who is extremely proactive and leaves no stone unturned in finding answers for her son, immediately searched the Internet and confirmed that AS seemed to describe Chris with remarkable accuracy. She found that her son's obliviousness to social cues, difficulty establishing friendships, obsessiveness, stiff affect, hypersensitivity, and awkwardness of movements all fell under the autism continuum.

But the symptom that we found most unusual when we began treating Chris was the sheer frequency of his hand washing. We prescribed *Syphilinum,* a homeopathic nosode that figures prominently in the literature for this habit. This medicine also covered the fixed nature of Chris' thoughts and behaviors.

No More Germ Stuff

Christopher's parents brought him back to our office two months later.

> *Big improvement. It took about a week for the medicine to act. Hand washing has dropped to a minimum. The ritual touching has stopped. Chris is able to listen much better, and is talking to other kids more. He got a star in class for keeping his hands to himself. Handwriting, drawing, and coloring are much more precise compared to the previous stick figures. Chris is showing more interest in his schoolwork, especially science. He's a bit nicer to his brother. The fear of the dark and the unknown are still there, but he's able now to put words to it. His voice has changed—less of a monotone and more modulation. His sense of humor is hugely different.*

Overall, Chris' parents were very pleased with the change. He was still loquacious with a tendency to obsess and perseverate, but less frequently and less intensely than before. Having read quite a bit more about AS, Chris' parents agreed that the diagnosis fit him well.

Four months after consulting us, Chris had progressed even further. His sensitivity to noise had improved for three months. The aggression and behavior had also been better until quite recently. His mother announced proudly that Chris was doing "unbelievably well" at school. Able to read at fourth-grade level, he was now getting along fine with the other kids. This was impressive, since the previous school year he was friendless and had been known to pin kids against the fence on a regular basis.

To his mom's amazement, feedback from Chris' teacher was positive: Chris was attentive, cooperative, participated appropriately in class activities, and would have had As if he had been in a graded classroom. This, his mother emphasized, was "a 180-degree turn-around from last year." The "germ stuff" was gone, hand washing was no longer an issue, and his handwriting was "light years better." Drawing, previously a slash-like scribble, continued to be precise and multicolored.

Further Progress
Chris continued to do well on the nosode for the first nine months of treatment. By that time, obsessiveness was not nearly as much of a concern. Sports skills were much improved, fears had diminished considerably, friends were not a problem, and his grades were fine. But there was still room for improvement on a number of fronts. Now his main challenges were excessive touching and pinching, yelling too much at his brother, and easily triggered irritability and impatience. Some other AS features also persisted, including stiff social interactions and speech, limited eye contact, and an exaggerated predisposition to follow rules to the letter.

We prescribed several different medicines that were given over the next two-and-a-half years. Overall Chris improved steadily, however, pressured by his teachers to improve Chris' focus in the classroom, his parents opted to also put him Concerta, a stimulant medication commonly used to treat ADD. It is not so common for parents to need to add psychotropic medications when the child is responding well to homeopathy, but it is understandable, when a particular area does not seem to be addressed, that parents may decide to also use a conventional medicine. The bottom line is to help the child be as happy and healthy as possible.

Chris continued to "cruise." A dynamite goalie on his soccer team, he became a fearless team member, not hesitating to "go for it" on the soccer field. This was a victory, whether or not his team won. Chris' mom remarked that he was doing "fabulously" in school. His social skills were "good, but formal." Although his parents were still satisfied with the youngster's progress, we believed there must be an even better medicine for him.

A Breakthrough

That winter, we spent two intensive weeks of homeopathic study in Mumbai (Bombay), India. By the next time we saw Chris, we had learned a new method of finding just the right medicine for him. When talking about Chris' fears, he confided:

> *I stopped watching Scooby Doo because there were lots of monsters. Some of them kept getting stuck in my head. Like the Yeti (the Abominable Snowman)... I knew it didn't exist, but I didn't believe that in my head. The feeling of the Yeti comes into my mind when I'm alone and in the dark. You know, they come out when you don't expect them. I feel like I'm on Scooby Doo and suddenly the Yeti comes out and chases me. It's an unexpected feeling that takes over my mind.*

The Yeti, and particularly the recurrent word "unexpected," caught our attention. The more we spoke with Chris, the more he used words like "unexpected" and "all of a sudden." He also generalized these phrases to describe other situations that frightened him. His underlying fear was that someone might be hiding somewhere and would suddenly grab him and start punching him. Not kill him, but "it would hurt a lot." Never before had we heard a youngster used the words "sudden" and "unexpected" so repeatedly.

Our ears perked up; we recognized these words as corresponding to a particular plant family of homeopathic medicines, and to a medicine that would not even have crossed our radar screen before attending the seminar in Mumbai. We prescribed *Oenanthe* (water hemlock). This plant belongs to the *Apiaceae* (also known as *Umbelliferae*, or celery) family, which has the theme of sudden blows or injuries, precisely Chris' fear.

To quote Chris' mom in the follow-up visit six weeks later:

Your remedy was incredible. He became a regular, taking-other-people's-feelings-into-consideration person. Forgive me while I gush. The holidays were marvelous. He was engaging in conversation instead of one-way talk. Chris had friends over and went to their houses throughout the vacation. He's trying new foods and activities. He'll actually eat chicken now. This is the best remedy so far in terms of making him fit into society better. He worked on a school project intensively for two weeks and ended up with the highest grade you could get. For a little ADHD kid, that was nothing short of a miracle.

Now it was Chris' turn to talk. What impressed us

right off was the change in his affect. His speech was relaxed and natural, not at all rigid or formal. We were amazed. Chris happily shared that he now had half a dozen friends. "Things aren't getting stuck in my head at night. No more Yetis. I forgot all about it." The remainder of our time together was spent with Chris babbling on about his new interest: *Star Wars*. We heard all about the Galactic Empire game, shield generators, and powerful weapons like air cruisers and destroyer droids.

Just a Regular Fourth Grader

Now, a year after we prescribed the *Oenanthe*, Chris' ability to express himself naturally and spontaneously has continued to improve. Honored as student of the month and a talented recorder player, Chris is also one of the better players on his baseball team. He can count seven friends, not bad for any kid, much less one diagnosed with AS and ADHD. Play dates and sleepovers are frequent. *Star Wars* continues to delight Chris, along with *Animal Crossing*. Chris is much kinder to and quieter with his brother, which pleases his parents to no end. According to Jenny:

> *It's as if the Asperger layers have peeled off and you can see who's under there. The most dramatic change started with what you gave him after you got back from India. He's made so many friends now that he's just a regular fourth grader. Folks who haven't seen Chris for a long time are dumbstruck!*

Gina: Flipping, Flapping, and Fidgeting

Gina was immature for a thirteen-year-old entering puberty. Physically, she was the size of an eight or nine-year-old. Developmental delay was evident by the time she was five, when her language abilities were assessed to be at the level of a three-year-old. The diagnosis was Pervasive Developmental Disorder (PDD).

Not blessed with an easy start in life, Gina was a C-section baby who cried from the moment she took her first breath outside the safety of the womb. She continued to awaken her weary parents with ear-piercing, inconsolable wails until she was three and a half. Comforting the child was to no avail. Immediately following her pertussis vaccine, Gina shrieked even louder and longer for a couple of days. As a toddler, Gina's tonsils were chronically enlarged and infected, disturbing her breathing during sleep, and leading to a tonsillectomy and adenoidectomy when she was six.

Gina's parents chose to home school her, supplemented with four hours a day of tutoring by an accredited teacher. The youngster experienced considerable difficulty with focusing, particularly with math, and her restlessness made it nearly impossible for Gina to remain in her seat and get her work done. The child had a habit of rocking in her seat, kicking her feet, or banging on the computer keyboard. Her attention span averaged fifteen seconds to a minute at the most. Easily distracted by noise, Gina had also been diagnosed with Central Auditory Processing Dsorder (CAPD). Though during infancy she was delighted to hear the sound of a vacuum cleaner, as she became older, it became intolerable.

Impulsive and impatient, Gina eventually got down to work only if her tutor persistently coaxed her to focus. The child thrived on one-on-one attention. No matter how hard she tried, Gina could not help but fidget, flap her hands, and chew on or flip her pencils. She exhibited a few obsessive tendencies, including lining up her toys and playing repetitively with string. Some of her favorite games involved removing and fiddling with shoelaces, twisting string, and tying knots.

Gina's mom complained that she chattered incessantly and tormented both mom and tutor with non-stop questions. The girl had an admirable thirst for learning; she just didn't want anyone to tell or show her how to do anything.

Dr. Pepper and the Disney Channel
If pushed too hard in schoolwork, Gina responded with neck jerking and grunting. These tics began after she was struck on the head by the trunk door of a friend's car, and worsened when taking Adderall and Concerta. Straterra, a non-stimulant medication for ADHD, did not aggravate the tics, but induced drowsiness. Tired of the side effects of conventional medications, his parents looked instead to homeopathic treatment, as is the case with many of our patients.

When it came to interests and hobbies, Gina's tastes were childish for a thirteen-year-old. For instance, she enjoyed simple picture books, and her favorite TV shows were on Nickelodeon and the Disney Channel. The youngster loved videos, except for scary ones. Computer savvy, Gina surfed the Net to research her favorite movies. Also high on her list of fun pastimes were going sailing with her dad and listening to Bible stories. A typical junk-food junkie, Gina loved popcorn, chocolate ice cream or pudding, lollipops, Dr. Pepper, and Coke.

Kind and Compassionate
Notably kind and compassionate, Gina demonstrated concern for others far beyond her years and was especially kind to those who were disabled. Gina wanted desperately to be around other kids, and to please prospective playmates, she was willing to go along with their

whims. She didn't have the best taste in friends and often ended up being the one to do all the giving. "I like kids who are younger or my age," Gina explained. "I wouldn't play with fifteen or sixteen-year-olds." She enjoyed hide and seek, running, and basketball, but found soccer too rough and confusing.

Special Features

 Gina was quite social compared to many children on the autism spectrum. Her main issues were developmental delay and emotional immaturity. She looked much younger than her age, preferred to play with children younger than herself, and lacked age-appropriate interests. Cognitive and academic progress were delayed. The child's mathematical ability was four or five years delayed. Gina could add and subtract, and was just starting to learn to count money. Due to visual processing impairment, writing was challenging, but she had no problem with typing.

We chose a medicine from the *Baryta* or barium group. Medicines made from this element, as mentioned in an earlier case, can typically benefit children who exhibit immaturity, dependence, timidity, and a tendency towards holding themselves back for fear of embarrassment. One of the lesser-known *Baryta* medicines, though, is known for working with patients who are more social and outgoing, and less timid. This medicine is *Baryta phosphoricum*. The phosphorus element adds sociability, kindness and compassion to the mix, as well as a strong desire for company, love, and acceptance. In Gina's case, we can see that she sought out friends and playmates, was sweet and kind, and was receptive to and giving of love and affection. Her childishness was a prominent feature and led her to choose younger children as playmates.

Follow-up Visits

At the first follow-up appointment, Gina's mother, Robin, was happy to say that her attention had improved, and that she no longer reacted to reprimands with nervous tics. Less fidgety and more attentive, she was doing better at her schoolwork, although impulsivity and loquacity were still concerns.

By the next visit, Gina had made a significant leap in growth, maturity and independence. Physical coordination and table manners were improved. The tics were completely gone except for one incidence of grunting after another child called her "retarded." (Gina's parents had never discussed with their daughter the diagnosis of PDD.)

Gina transformed even more after the second dose of the same medicine. Four months later, Robin bubbled, "Gina seems smarter. She read *three* chapters of a SpongeBob book at a sitting. Her coordination is better, and she's not obsessed with strings anymore. Gina grew an inch within a week of taking the last dose, and her breasts seemed to have grown a bit." The rocking and tics had stopped entirely. Robin described the change over the previous four months as "night and day." Gina was not nearly as stressed, and the family found her much easier to be around. Both Robin and the tutor reported that learning came more easily, and that the child was more open to constructive criticism. Gina told us how much fun she had at overnight camp. The counselors had marveled at her compassion towards the handicapped children at the camp. The girl had made new friends and had been invited to and hosted sleepovers. Gina even showed less interest in candy, choosing instead hot dogs, steak, and pizza.

Over the following months, the child continued to be on a sharp maturation curve. Robin reported, "She's doing better than ever before. Gina is even talking about what she'll do when she grows up." Gina was able to think more clearly and to answer questions and solve problems more quickly. All who know her are favorably impressed with the positive changes they have noticed in Gina since beginning homeopathy.

Paolo: Free Trogs and Cracknutters

Paolo, eight years old, was adopted from a Brazilian orphanage.. A charmer from the get-go, everyone who met the child was mesmerized by his contagious smile and liquid brown eyes. With strangers, Paolo was quite gregarious. At home, he was the opposite—cranky, complaining, and constantly dissatisfied.

Paolo's mom recounted how a "demon look" would come over his face, at which time he would behave as if he were drunk. During these episodes, Paolo would roll his eyes wildly, run around frenetically, and literally bounce off the walls. The child's outbursts were even more extreme after ingesting food colorings, additives and preservatives. This marked correlation had led his mother to put him on the Feingold diet, which had clearly helped to some degree. One particular afternoon, Paolo, unbeknownst to his mother, had pilfered some food-coloring-laden candy in the supermarket. That evening, in church, he sang and whistled for an hour straight. His parents' reproaches didn't faze him in the least. Rebellious against his restricted diet, Paolo ate any "forbidden" food he could get his hands on.

Paolo's incessant "whys" exhausted even the patience of an adoring mother. After he would ask "What is Paolo doing?" five or ten times, though the answer was quite obvious, his mother would finally gave in and tell him. Rather than being content with her answer, the interrogation now switched to, "Why is Paolo doing it?" Instead of using "I" when referring to himself, he often began his sentences with his own name, referring to himself in the third person: "Paolo wants to go to the store today." Dyslexic, the boy routinely mixed up words and phrases and reversed letters, even whole words—"free trog" instead of "tree frog", "Acrifa" for "Africa", "cracknutter" for "nutcracker", and "lawn the mow" instead of "mow the lawn".

Talk About the Leopard I Am

Paolo loved to torment the family cat by grabbing her from behind or frightening her with sticks. The cat knew to steer clear of him, especially if he was in one of his strange moods. Paolo also loved to pretend he was an animal. Whenever he saw an animal, either in real life or in a book or video, Paolo became that creature, and begged his parents to share, in explicit detail, everything they knew about that kind of animal. "Talk about the leopard I am. Tell me his name and what he eats for dinner." When he first arrived from Brazil, he ate his food from a dish on the floor, just like their kitty.

Other unusual mannerisms included swiveling his head from side to side and sucking his thumb while rolling on the floor. The youngster had the habit of touching and smelling everything he picked up. He also insisted that his mother take both parts of their conversations, and that she say aloud certain phrases just as he instructed.

Paolo was not much interested in going outside, though he occasionally threw his baseball bat around the yard or played briefly on the swing. Even inside, it was hard for the child to find an activity he enjoyed. Drawing and coloring were no fun. Only videos or listening to books read to him by his parents held the boy's interest for very long. Paolo liked being with other children, but they avoided him. Consequently, Paolo had no one he could call a friend.

Bob the Builder and Hot Dogs, Cool Cats

More than willing to participate in the homeopathic interview, Paolo immediately contradicted his mother by assuring us that he had plenty of friends, and loved playing outside. He also described how much he liked building towers with blocks, then knocking them down for fun. He enjoyed his *Bob the Builder* video, because "Bob was a worker, who had a machine and built with wood". Another favorite video was *Hot Dogs, Cool Cats*. In fact, Paolo admitted his affinity for all kinds of animals—cats, squirrels, bunnies, leopards and parakeets. He liked to play hide and seek with his cat, Thomas, and in quiet moments, drew pictures of the kitty. "Thomas is the bravest cat I've ever met!" exclaimed Paolo.

Paolo was an active child. He was always twisting himself in the phone cord, or rolling in the car, across the floor, or in bed. Thumb sucking and drooling were also frequent, as were spinning, banging, and crashing into whatever obstacles were in his way. Paolo also had the habit of spinning his toys. Even during quiet play, Paolo would mutter with agitation and make random threats like "I'll hit you and put you in jail."

Reaction to an MMR Vaccine

One possible source of Paolo's developmental and social delay was a severe reaction to the MMR vaccine at twenty-seven months, shortly after he was adopted. The boy immediately developed an inflamed lump on his buttocks, and limped around irritably for days. Afterwards Paolo was far more upset than before the immunization and screamed inconsolably. The shrieking continued with frequency throughout his toddler-hood. Paolo lost nearly two years of language development, and his motor skills and balance declined as well. He lost any knowledge of how to play and, if given toys, would simply not know what to do with them. Prior to the immunization, despite having been raised in an orphanage, the boy's development appeared normal. Actually, Paolo had been the darling of the orphanage, so much so that he had been given a crib with a view!

Special Features

 Paolo's developmental delay and autistic features may have resulted from a couple of factors. An orphan of uncertain parentage, the family history of the birth parents is not available. However, it is clear that the boy suffered a severe reaction to the MMR vaccine. His "intoxicated" behavior and demon-like demeanor were clearly exacerbated by food additives. In addition to these features, Paolo was fascinated with being an animal and was severely dyslexic.

We prescribed for Paolo the homeopathic medicine derived from chocolate. One of the main characteristics of youngsters needing this particular medicine is their animal-like tendencies. Another indication for *Chocolate* is a feeling of abandonment and a desire for extra love and attention, as is often seen in orphans. These kids feel as if they missed out on the nurturing and fun of infancy and childhood. Youngsters needing this medicine can make mistakes in speaking or writing and may act or feel as though they were intoxicated.

More Affectionate than Ever Before

Paolo benefited a great deal from the *Chocolate*. At first, he experienced a brief return of symptoms from the past, a common phenomenon after being given the correct medicine. These included an episode of hysterical crying and regression reminiscent of his behavior two years earlier. For a week or two, Paolo hid under the table when he was angry, as he had done around the same time as the wailing. Everything settled down after the initial couple of weeks. Paolo's mom reported at his six-week return visit, "On the whole, he is better than before. He is easier to get along with and more cooperative. The good far outweighs the bad."

The most startling change was Paolo's spontaneous affection. Much to his parents' delight, he was more cuddly and sweeter than they had ever seen him. The "drunk behavior" and "demon look" had also disappeared. The kitty must have breathed a sigh of relief, because Paolo now merely chased her playfully rather than tormenting her. The twirling and spinning had stopped as well.

The youngster's drawing abilities had improved significantly, especially cats, dinosaurs, and zebras. To his parents' amazement, Paolo stopped repeating the same questions over and over, though he still asked "why?" a number of times in a series. Paolo's speech and writing were better as well, and he no longer reversed words and letters. Another interesting change was that he no longer referred to himself in the third person. Paolo still sucked his thumb and rolled around, though less frequently than before taking the *Chocolate*. He still loved to pretend he was a lion, a bear, or a tiger, and continued to beg his parents to describe the animal he was portraying.

The Diagnosis of PDD-NOS No Longer Fit
With the stress of school starting, Paolo suffered a partial return of his symptoms, which homeopaths call a "relapse," and we repeated the medicine. Unfortunately, that dose did not act, possibly because of a conventional

medication given to the boy for ringworm. We gave a stronger dose of the *Chocolate*. Within an hour after taking the dose, Paolo was "a different child." He soon fully recovered all the gains he had made previously, and more.

Two months later he received another dose after being exposed to strong incense at church. Once again he responded beautifully to the medicine. Paolo's teacher confirmed that he was staying on task and following directions well. He still reacted occasionally to offending foods, such as candy with food coloring, but his reactions were less frequent and less severe.

Paolo has continued to progress extremely well over the past year, with occasional repetitions of the *Chocolate*. He has also become increasingly affectionate and cooperative. A developmental pediatrician concluded that, although the child was previously diagnosed with Pervasive Developmental Disability-Not Otherwise Spec-ified (PDD-NOS), Paolo's symptoms fit AS better. But given how well he related to adults and peers, he felt that even that diagnosis was no longer quite ap-propriate.

9

Sensitive and Selective
Picky in a Prickly World

Many children with ASD struggle with sensory integration, and their sensitivities can greatly interfere with their daily routine. When the brain in unable to adequately filter sensory information, it can misinterpret the strength of the stimulus. A child can be either over- or under-responsive to sensory stimuli such as touch, taste, sound or scent. A child with ASD who is over-responsive may develop sensory defensiveness, avoiding sounds, tastes, textures, touch, and smells that an NT wouldn't give a second thought. A child who is under-responsive may seek more intense sensations or sensory experiences of an extended duration. Some ASD kids are both over- and under-responsive; for example, needing to twirl and constantly "bouncing off the walls," but being unable to tolerate certain food textures or a scratchy collar.

For an oversensitive child with ASD, a mall, a noisy classroom, or even the flush of a toilet may be an uncomfortable, or painful, auditory experience. Likewise, someone with a tactile sensitivity may experience a shirt tag or particular cloth textures as utterly unbearable. Or, having his hair brushed or cut can feel like torture.

Such sensitivies can extend to food preferences as well. This is referred to as oral defensiveness. The carbonated fizz of a soda pop may create palpable discomfort. Foods with unusual textures, such as the dry crunch of a cracker or pretzel or the gooeyness of chocolate pudding, may be perceived as unpleasant. His sense of smell may also be extremely sensitive, causing a child with ASD to run from the house if someone is cooking bacon or cabbage or burning toast. As a result, many of these kids are extremely picky eaters and a terrific challenge for parents to feed. In an attempt to accommodate the child's sensory needs, the parents' patience and creativity are often severely put to the test.

Fortunately, homeopathy can be extremely helpful in reducing these exaggerated sensitivities. The cases in this chapter illustrate how the correct homeopathic medicine can make a world of difference for a child with sensory integration issues.

Cody: **Too Sensitive for Words**

We were just about to leave for Switzerland to present an ADHD seminar to professional homeopaths when we received an e-mail message from Cody's mother asking for help. An American living in Italy, his mom had read *Ritalin-Free Kids* and very much wanted us to treat her two children. She was willing to do the consultations by phone, but was overjoyed to hear we were on our way to Europe. Unfortunately, Cody's mom already had a trip to the United States planned for that time, so his dad brought him and his sister to Zurich to see us.

Cody's dad cut to the chase:

> *Cody has a problem with sensory overload. If you say too much to him for too long, he simply throws his hands over his ears. He just can't take it. He breaks down and starts crying. Cody screams at the*

*top of his lungs for no apparent reason. It is like his
emotions hit a boiling point and he spews them all
out. When he goes into one of those tirades, there's
nothing you can do to make him feel better.*

From the time he was a toddler to age five, Cody
developed a high fever and inconsolable crying after each
round of immunizations. His reactions were so severe
that his mom refused to allow the children to be immu-
nized again. Ear infections had been a recurrent problem
when Cody was younger, perhaps because he was
switched to formula after having been breastfed for five
months. Later he suffered from asthma, as did his older
brother. Bright beyond his years, Cody had skipped from
kindergarten to second grade. His peers belittled him,
and he suffered terribly from the derision. The first
words out of Cody's mouth upon arriving home from
school were, "They think my ideas are stupid," at which
point he would sigh heavily and break into sobs.
Risperdal, an antipsychotic medication used off-label
with children to control difficult behaviors and mitigate
moods, resulted in a twenty-pound weight gain. Now, in
addition to being the youngest kid in his class (eight years
old and in the third grade), Cody was obese and clumsy.
Any physical exertion caused him discomfort and to
become overheated.

Cody and his older brother were both diagnosed
with AS. His dad's words were reminiscent of what we
hear so often from parents of children with AS: "It's like
he marches to the beat of a different drummer. It might
not be the time or place to do it socially. Cody's kind of
in his own little world."

Cody was certainly not a demanding child. Capable
of entertaining himself with video games or books, Cody
often disappeared to "do his own thing." Although very

intelligent, the youngster's grades were only average. Without Risperdal, Cody would "rant and rave and be set off by the smallest thing," such as his sister touching him. It didn't take much at all for him to "go off the deep end." When unmedicated, Cody blew up daily, a trait his dad referred to as "a short fuse." For example, if his dad came home from work and, in a normal tone of voice, told Cody to go do his homework, the boy might react by throwing his book bag, insisting vociferously that he was *not* going to do his homework, raising his hands to his face, and falling into heart-wrenching sobs. Once the lid blew off, there was no consoling Cody and no reasoning with him. The ensuing thirty minutes consisted of Cody's muttering under his breath and slamming doors.

Video games were a serious matter for this young man. Losing was not an option. When it looked like he was not going to win, Cody would throw the game to the floor and burst into tears. According to his dad, "We're here because we're starting to get complaints from school that Cody is disruptive in class. It's his emotional outbursts. The school psychologist wants him to stay on Risperdal, and his mother and I would like to have him off of it. I know, when I was a kid, I was a hellion. So were my brothers and sisters. But we weren't drugged, doped up, and drooling."

A Lot Like His Older Brother

His brother, Dennis, was diagnosed first with ADD, then Asperger's. And now, Cody. In the grand scheme of things, I think his real problem is dealing with his emotions in a way that is socially acceptable. Cody is a real sensitive guy. One night, as I got home late from work, I found Cody bawling. 'It's sooo cute,' he cooed. He was going gaga over one of the teddy bears in my wife's collection that had just come in the mail. Cody went on for an hour sobbing heavily about how adorable it was. He just couldn't contain it. Those are the kind of outbursts I mean. It can be over something sad or happy or just out of frustration.

Neither one of the boys is much into athletics. They don't climb trees or run or play ball. They don't interact well with others. Dennis didn't have friends till he was thirteen.

Before I left for the Middle East, Cody and I were buds. When I returned after seven months of active duty, our relationship wasn't the same. It was true for Dennis, too. They kiss their mom good-night, but not me. To this day, if there's a problem they go to her rather than me. It didn't used to be like that.

Cody's hearing tested normal. I think it's just sensory overload. He has to dash out of the class-room if the noise is too much for him. Being touched by strangers puts him over the top. He just flinches. It's as if you're invading his personal space. And Cody's pain threshold is way low. Before, he totally freaked out when we took him to the dentist. He's still skittish about going. Having his blood drawn is traumatic. Cody yelled and squealed after he threw up with a flu—it was almost a panic reaction. I had a hard time calming him down. I'd say his level of sensitivity is about eight out of ten.

Smells are tough for him, too. The odor of peanuts is unbearable. He's over-the-top picky about food. He hates tomato sauce and sugar. Cody can't stand noise and lights or someone brushing up against him. And chaotic situations with too much activity or visual stimuli. I'd call it a fear of over-stimulation.

An Exquisite Sensitivity to Needles

Cody was delightfully communicative. First we discussed his favorite video games, a typical lead-in we use to break the ice with children during the initial interview. Then Cody shared with us how hard it was for him to concentrate because a classmate made so much noise. When annoyed by noise at home, Cody would retreat to his room and play *Nintendo* or *Game Cube.*

The youngster continued to describe the nature of his sensitivities:

> *When I hear loud noise, it feels like a bunch of arrows going into my eardrums. The pain is like needles. And my face is sensitive, too. The last time I tripped during recess, my face dragged on the sharp ground. It's a good thing I didn't scrape my eyes. My whole body is sensitive. Sometimes I get smacked on my hand and it feels like a bunch of splinters going into it. Like my hand is made of wood.*
>
> *When I go to the dentist and get drilled, it's like there's electricity coming right out of my mouth. Like an electric shock. When the dentist gives Novocaine, it feels like a giant arrow going into my gum. And when people step on me, it feels like a million needles going into my foot. God, it hurts! Or when somebody at school smacks me or punches me. My whole body can feel like that. Oh, God! When people tease me, I just want to beat them up. Kids who threaten me and say they're gonna beat me up or kill me. And they curse at me. It happens very often. Some people are not very nice to me when I want them to be nice.*

Cody complained that his sister would scratch his arm until it nearly bled. "It was cut open, well, not exactly cut open because her nails weren't sharp enough. And she used to bite me!" With Cody, everything was about being pierced or poked.

About Arrows, Swords, and Anvils

Few patients, adult or child, are as in touch with and articulate about their peculiar sensitivities as Cody. One of the keys homeopaths use to unlock the door of the subconscious to better understand our patients is to inquire about interests and hobbies, fears, and dreams. These can give us valuable clues that can help lead us to the best medicine for the child. Cody loved to cook, especially Italian and French cuisine. He particularly enjoyed speaking in an Italian accent while he prepared meals. "Even if it's French food, I say, 'Mama mia!' "

When we inquired about fears, perhaps you can guess Cody's response:

I'm really scared of hornets. They're huge. About as big as my hand. Really huge. I've seen them on TV. I'm also afraid of starfish because they suck on you. In fact, when I see one, I feel like getting a shotgun and shooting it. You know, starfish sometimes crawl up on my hand and suck on it and won't get off. And ticks. Because they bite you. I really hate that! And I really friggin' hate blood! It scares me so much that I want to pass out. Blood mostly scares me because of how much the pain hurts when I bleed.

Initially, Cody complained that he was "sick and tired of telling people my dreams," but his reluctance was short-lived.

I had this wonderful dream where I had a sword case with a big sword and I started bashing people with it. I liked to cut them and other things in the dream. I just like doing because it was fun—swinging the sword and cutting things. I was also shooting arrows. Regular arrows, fire arrows, and light arrows with a golden crystal.

When we asked Cody if there were anything he would like to change about his life, replied, "I'd change everything into magic. Be the emperor of the world. I'd be the half emperor and half warrior. Be the emperor for a little while, then go out in the world and fight people because I like to go on adventures and kill the people who beat me up. I'd kill them, maybe with a sword."

Finally, we questioned Cody about his recurrent headaches. Again, we were amazed by his ability to describe the pain so vividly: "It's kind of like there's a giant anvil on my brain. Being crushed by a giant anvil. Like it's crushing my head. Turning, rotating, going up and down. That's what the anvil feels like on my head."

Exceptional Features

 You don't have to be a homeopath to be able to identify what stands out most about Cody. The primary issue of patients needing homeopathic medicines made from plants is sensitivity. There is no question that this was the case with Cody. His specific sensitivity was to being injured by anything sharp. His definition of sharp extended beyond needles, knives, arrows, hornets, and fingernails, to objects we do not routinely consider sharp, such as starfish or playground gravel. This hypersensitivity expressed itself even in Cody's dream life. One plant family that is indicated for those sensitive to pain is the *Loganaceaes*. The specific medicine Cody needed was *Spigelia,* or pinkroot. The best known features of children needing this medicine are the extreme fear of needles and sharp, pointed objects as well as migraine headaches that feel like a sharp, red hot poker piercing the left eye. It was fascinating to hear Cody explain so clearly just how sensitive he was. It might be quite difficult for someone not as exquisitely sensitive to comprehend this heightened sensitivity, particularly a callous schoolyard bully.

Moods, Headaches, and Sensitivity All Improve

We typically schedule the first follow-up appointment six weeks after the medicine is administered. Cody's mom was not able to give him the *Spigelia* until one month after we saw him, and his first follow-up telephone consultation was delayed until five months later. Cody had responded well for several months: more cooperative in school, less vulgar, no headaches. Then his behavior began to deteriorate. We wished his mother had communicated with us earlier, because we would have promptly repeated the medicine when this deterioration started. Following another dose of *Spigelia,* Cody again improved for a couple of months, though his response was somewhat confused by a Risperdal dosage change, which resulted in a forty-pound weight gain!

The response to the higher dose of the homeopathic medicine was even more dramatic. The youngster was now better able to get along with other children. Despite having discontinued the Risperdal, his irritability had diminished considerably, and he was back to his "sweet, lovable" self. "Most of the time he's just a very sweet soul," his dad said. The headaches had not returned, the episodes of sensitivity were far less frequent, and Cody no longer dreamed of hurting other children. He no longer experienced the splinter-like sensation in his face, the fear of hornets was less, and Cody no longer screamed at the sight of a knife. Now, a year after beginning treatment, Cody continues to do well, has been off the Risperdal for six months, and his clothing size has dropped from an eighteen to a twelve.

Kevin: The Verbatim Kid

Kevin, six years old, had a number of features that stood out. For example, he was an agile gymnast who could perform amazing antics. He was a veritable wizard at feeding back video dialogue word for word. Kevin always had to have something in his mouth. He would chew his fingers, zippers, and rubber tags. It didn't seem to matter what the objects were, as long as Kevin had *something* in his mouth to chew on. His teeth were ground down so severely that no enamel remained. By the time we met Kevin by phone, eight of his molars had already been capped!

Extremely noise sensitive, the boy particularly disliked one television show in which the star spoke quickly in a hard, staccato. Upon hearing that voice, Kevin would clasp both hands over his ears and scream, "Turn it off!" The whirring noise of fans running at high speed was also intolerable to Kevin. But Kevin was quite a music fan, his tastes ranging from blues to U2, two-step to jive. And was Kevin rhythmic! He had the Elvis hip swish down to an art. But it had to be music that he liked. Led Zeppelin or KISS would send Kevin racing to the other end of the house. Sometimes he would make loud noises himself, despite his sensitivity to them.

Not good with "why" questions, Kevin was better at concrete thinking than abstractions. He didn't last long playing pretend games with other children. Ten to fifteen seconds of playing in the toy kitchen was enough for him. The concept seemed to go over his head, and he was off to something else. Ninety percent of the boy's play was parallel rather than interactive. The other children may as well have been in another room for all the attention Kevin gave them.

Yet the child loved being touched and cuddled. He was almost too trusting; he would talk to anyone just to have a connection. He was the same way with animals—Kevin would fearlessly amble up to strange dogs. The more a dog barked at him, the more he thought it was hilarious. His mom described it as a lack of street smarts.

A Challenging Entry into Life

Kevin's mom, Susan, wondered, when pregnant with Kevin, if something were wrong with her fetus. "He just wasn't a mover like his sister." She had been quite ill with a gastrointestinal flu during the pregnancy, and was treated with *Belladonna* in a synthetic, rather than homeopathic, form. The birth was traumatic: the cord was wrapped around the baby's neck so Susan had to stop pushing. He was delivered three days past the due date and weighed a whopping nine pounds. Kevin's APGAR score was only a six, so oxygen was administered.

Susan struggled with breastfeeding, and Kevin was diagnosed with failure to thrive, resulting in supplementation with formula. Constipation was a problem from birth, to which Susan responded by giving Kevin corn syrup. Adding to the challenge, his parents needed to double diaper Kevin due to his hip dysplasia. To her credit, Susan persevered, and continued with some breastfeeding until Kevin turned four. Susan felt that he became markedly more delayed around the age of four. His playschool teacher then recommended that he receive testing, and he was diagnosed with AS.

Spinning, Spirited, and Special Needs

Susan described her son as "fun-loving, easy-going, and quite a talker." He reveled in reciting back whatever he heard on TV, rehearsing the lines to make sure they came out just right. A jumper, dancer, and climber, Kevin enjoyed spinning in chairs and hoisting himself onto a chair to retrieve apple juice from the refrigerator, adamantly resisting assistance. A wandering mind made it difficult for him to keep his attention on one conversation or activity. This little guy could also rage, tensing his body, assuming a fighting stance, clenching his teeth, and yelling angrily, "Don't do that! I don't like it!"

Concepts were tough for Kevin. It was difficult for him to grasp that "Susan" and "his mom" could be the same person. His verbal communication skills were limited, so his parents relied on body language to interpret his likes and dislikes. By eleven months Kevin uttered only basic words such as "Dada." Eye contact was minimal. Fine motor skills were limited, although hand-eye coordination was very good. Kevin learned more easily with hands-on skills such as assembling puzzles. Kevin was unable to learn his own name until the age of four and a half years. In new situations or around people with whom he felt ill at ease, Kevin's *modus operandi* was avoidance.

Kevin had other traits reminiscent of children with AS. He loved books, insisting on reading and rereading the same ones over and over. Finicky about foods and textures, Kevin hated apples and bananas, and was revolted by touching gooey stuff such as shaving cream and Play-doh®. He was highly sensitive to having his hair brushed, combed, or pulled. There was forever something in Kevin's mouth whenever he felt stressed, especially the first two fingernails of each hand. He also suffered from cold sores during these times. We weren't able to gather much information directly from Kevin because, though animated and friendly, his attention span for our phone conversation was ten seconds flat. His personal record for conversational endurance had been set the previous week, talking with his aunt for a full five minutes.

Exceptional Features

 We initially prescribed *Theridion* for Kevin, the spider medicine mentioned previously as helpful for overly sensitive, highly active children, especially those with a high degree of sensitivity to noise. The combination of the boy's gymnastic ability, love of music, rhythmic talent, and excruciating sensitivity to noise are consistent with this medicine. Despite a favorable response to the *Theridion*, however, one year into treatment we found a medicine that suited him better.

We found it notable that Kevin's mom, Susan, was medicated with *Belladonna* during the pregnancy. The medicine came to our attention again when it produced an effective response in Kevin during an acute fever, as well as at the onset of migraine headaches. Though both *Theridion* and *Belladonna* had unquestionable effect on Kevin, the *Belladonna* has produced a more dramatic result. It's likely that the administration of the plant in medicinal form during the pregnancy sensitized him to need it homeopathically.

Better All Around

Susan and Kevin were able to come to Seattle for a visit one month after beginning homeopathic care, so we could finally meet them in person. Within the first month of treatment, Kevin was verbalizing more, exhibiting a faster response time, and speaking in more complete sentences. Nose picking, which Susan had forgotten to mention during our initial phone consultation, had decreased. Kevin was no longer peering in every mirror that he passed to make strange faces. Kevin was making more of an effort to interact with other children, though still not age appropriately. He could also tolerate his mother playing with his hair, which was impossible before treatment, and his noise tolerance had improved. The boy's habitual chewing and temper outbursts were unchanged. Susan mentioned that Kevin had suffered from heat stroke during a recent hot spell.

Over the next several months, Kevin became less prone to angry outbursts, his tripping diminished, and he continued to use more words. His reading skills "skyrocketed." Kevin began to ask "why?" and "when?" and stayed more on topic, rather than answering irrelevantly. His pronunciation blossomed, and he appeared generally more aware of what was going on. The child became more willing to do his schoolwork. The spinning ceased, nail-biting decreased, and his other self-stimulatory behaviors were less frequent. Also, his episodes of cold sores were infrequent.

It was during this period that Kevin had a high fever that his mother self-treated successfully with a dose of homeopathic *Belladonna*. After this, she noticed that his memory, eye contact, and listening skills improved, and his reading skills "had picked up like crazy." Nine months after treatment, Kevin's parents estimated his overall improvement to be 80%. His reading had jumped from a second-grade level to a fifth-grade level during that period. Kevin was now developing a delightful sense of humor and a twinkle in his eye.

A Better Match

Kevin's mom reported a new fear: the dark. A night-light was now mandatory for him to go to sleep. In addition,

Kevin had developed a fear of certain movies because they were too scary. It was at this point that Susan mentioned she had given Kevin a dose of homeopathic *Belladonna* for a migraine, a new symptom. The head pain was severe and accompanied by vomiting. Kevin lamented that his head "was killing him" and that he wanted to die. A low dose of *Belladonna*, given once, took care of the head pain and put Kevin right to sleep.

We inquired further about possible *Belladonna* symptoms at this time, knowing that patients needing both *Theridion* and *Belladonna* can have a number of symptoms in common, especially the keen sensitivity to noise. A child's response to a particular homeopathic medicine prescribed for clear acute symptoms can lead a homeopath to change medicines. Susan shared that Kevin became hot, red-faced, and clammy after exerting himself for an hour out in the sun. His cheeks, she added, turned bright red. We recalled the increased sensitivity of the scalp, another typical *Belladonna* symptom. Now, when asked about it, Susan confirmed that Kevin used to flinch whenever his nails were cut and that his face was very flushed with the migraine (also characteristic of people needing *Belladonna*). So, we gave Kevin a higher dose of homeopathic *Belladonna* than his mother had administered from her home kit.

90% Better and Still Improving
Since changing to *Belladonna*, Kevin's progress has been even more consistent and dramatic. The self-stimulatory behavior has occurred only once. There have been no headaches, and no more hands over the ears when Kevin is around noise. Sensitivity to the sun has decreased, despite spending more time outside during the summer. Hair combing and washing were no longer an ordeal. Kevin learned to dive underwater with his eyes open.

This was quite a change; previously he had avoided water on his face, a feature his mother had never mentioned. Kevin's dread of water was another important confirmatory symptom of *Belladonna*.

It has been 15 months since Kevin began taking the *Belladonna* and 28 months since we first started treating him. Although the course of homeopathic treatment is by no means finished, his parents estimate the improvement at 85-90%. They still have a live-in TV announcer. Kevin has the special talent of memorizing *TV Guide* cover to cover after reading it just once. His dad jokes, "It's a good thing we don't have cable!" Kevin and his dad recently returned from a problem-free overnight Boy Scout trip. During our last phone consultation, Susan chuckled, "Sometimes Kevin has really deep thoughts. Like the other day when he remarked, 'Mom, you have a lot to learn about me. I'm very impressed with your hard job of learning about my world.'"

Conner: Clawing, Biting, Swearing, and Screaming

Michelle was very much looking forward to our treating her seven-year-old son, Conner. She explained privately,

Conner's dad and I fought a lot during the pregnancy. Having him was the only reason we stayed together. During the first and second trimesters, I was in a constant adrenaline rush. My basic feeling was one of being trapped. I found myself in a situation I could not get out of. The family violence continued when Conner was an infant and toddler. There was always shouting and throwing things. Now and then his dad hit me. We're in the midst of an ugly divorce now. I've been trying to shield Conner and his sister from what's going on.

It's Conner's rage that brings me here. We've been doing the Feingold Diet with some benefit, but his temper is still out of control. I can say something unimportant to him, and it's as if a little switch goes on, especially if he's tired or hungry. Suddenly he's screaming, clawing, biting, and leaving welts on my skin. Out of the blue, this kid goes from being mildly frustrated to a cornered animal. It's like putting a cat in a basket. If there's one thing that Conner hates, it's being held down. If you restrain him, he'll bite. Then, when you release him, he'll hit you. The trigger might be an event Conner perceives as unfair, or even tripping over something on the floor, or a meltdown after being teased. He becomes livid, sinks his teeth into my shoulder as I try to pick him up, and threatens to pull out my eyes.

Conner's behavior was even worse before we started the Feingold Diet. All hell broke lose every day. Over the past four years, he's attended seven different schools and daycares. There was no way I could take him to a neighbor's, and he never got invited to other kids' houses. On a typical day back then, Conner would come home from preschool and dissolve into a tantrum at the least thing.

Conner would insist vehemently that his parents couldn't make him do anything he didn't want to do. These power struggles usually ended with one of them dragging him to his room, kicking and screaming. On a number of occasions during these meltdowns, Conner bit hard enough to break the skin. There was no way his parents could touch or hold him until he had calmed down on his own.

The previous year, he had gotten in big trouble at school for calling his teacher the F-word and trying to push her down a flight of stairs. And that was only kindergarten! The second day of school, he demanded of his teacher, "Get out of my way!" Often rude and insolent, he simply did not know when to stop. Other children did not appreciate his coming furtively behind them and stretching his shirt over their heads, grabbing things from them, or knocking off their glasses. Seven-year-old Conner's tantrums, replete with, kicking, biting, swearing, and scratching, were much worse than those of his two-year-old sister.

Terrified With Violent Reactions

Clothing that was too tight or that rubbed him uncomfortably was intolerable. He flat out rejected shirts or pants that had ever caught a burr in the bushes. From the age of three, Conner refused to wear socks, and he could not stand having his nails cut. Highly sensitive to particular foods, Conner reacted violently to Skittles, and exhibited muscle jerking after eating even a single Ritz cracker.

Unwilling to go to sleep without his mom lying beside him, the boy would only sleep in her bed. Nor would he go upstairs alone, even for a minute, even if all the lights were on. He had recently become "petrified of dogs," though the family had always had a large dog.

When Conner was tiny, I would hold him tightly while his father yelled at me, punched the wall, and threw things. At three or four he would run between us, pounding his fists on our legs shouting 'Don't fight!' Conner seemed especially affected one time when his father was in my face, shaking my shoulders. After that, as soon as voices were raised, even in laughter, Conner hid immediately.

At nineteen months, Conner was hospitalized for dehydration after a bad flu. When they tried to start an IV to give him fluids, the medical staff refused to allow his dad and me to be in the room. They had to do three pokes in one arm and four in the next because his veins kept collapsing. Conner was strapped down, screaming. The staff would not permit me to breastfeed him and tried to keep me away from him so he wouldn't want to nurse. I battled with them for 24 hours straight.

There was another incident that seemed to terrify Conner. I had a full-term stillborn daughter when Conner was just shy of four. Right after the baby was born, my husband burst into uncontrollable animal-like sobbing. Conner became extremely frightened by his dad's howling. I don't think he's ever completely gotten over that. Before, he'd been an agreeable, if stubborn, toddler. It was shortly afterward that the raging tantrums really started.

I Don't Like Being Held Tight

When we asked Conner if anything bothered him, he replied straightforwardly, "I don't like being held tight. It's not fun. You just try to get away." He went on to share that he was a bit afraid of dark. It felt to him like being blindfolded.

When his mother mentioned to us that he'd been having bad dreams about yellow-headed kidnappers lately, Conner spit at her, explaining, "I spit when I try to keep you from attacking me," at which point he buried his head deeply in the chair. His mood quickly turned nasty, first ordering his mother to move her feet off the floor and sit in a particular chair. Then the youngster proceeded to run away from her, spitting, and adamantly refusing to cooperate. Michelle continued:

Conner has always hated getting water splashed on him, especially on his face and head. As a baby, washing his hair was challenging because he would squirm and try to get away. Even a wet washcloth on his head was objectionable.

Even now, in new situations, Conner reacts by closing his eyes, flopping his head around, and screaming in a high, squeaky voice. Eye contact has been difficult for him from the start. Conner doesn't seem to grasp where his body ends and the other children's bodies begin. He prefers rough and tumble play like bouncing off the trampoline, crashing spaceships into other objects, or jumping on another child.

Exceptional Features

Conner's biting, spitting, clawing, and threatening suggested a homeopathic medicine made from an animal, as did the intense victim-aggressor relationship between his parents. Or perhaps one of the homeopathic plant medicines, such as those in the *Solanaceae* (nightshade) family that share many characteristics with animal medicines. Observing the interaction between Conner and Michelle in our office during his angry outburst reminded us of cats and dogs; dogs also terrified him.

Overall, Conner's most extreme sensitivity was to being restrained, reminiscent of his mom's trapped feeling while pregnant with him. When Conner was restrained in any way, his response was to bite, flail, and to try to find a way out, just like a wild animal.

We first prescribed *Stramonium*, and saw some improvement. We observed still further improvement after switching to another medicine, *Lyssin*. But our final choice of a medicine extracted from peregrine falcon proved, by far, to be the most effective remedy for Conner.

Rabid Rage

Five weeks after he took the *Stramonium*, Conner's fears were less intense, he was no longer having nightmares, and his fear of dogs had lessened somewhat. *Stramonium*, given at two-month intervals, benefited Conner to some extent over the next eight months. Until the dose wore off each time, the tantrums were considerably better, and the biting diminished. As long as the medicine was acting, Conner was willing to sleep alone in his own bed; when it stopped acting, he reverted to insisting on sleeping with Michelle. We were not satisfied with the amount of improvement, though.

We restudied Conner's case and, based on his rage, fear of water, animal-like behavior, and terror of dogs, prescribed *Lyssin*. At his next appointment three months later, we learned that Conner had recently made a surprisingly smooth transition from a small, private classroom to a public school. Hitting was less, biting was gone, and Conner was "hugely better with water, willing to lay down in the bathtub and gets his hair wet for the first time in his life." His speech therapist was particularly impressed with his progress, as was the sand-tray therapist who had been seeing Conner for two years. She had observed such a significant changes in the boy that she had recently "fired him" from therapy.

Over the next year, Conner's progress continued. On those occasions when Conner did experience a meltdown, it was short-lived and he could recover quickly. The ability to back down was a new skill for him. Michelle also reported "a dramatic improvement socially." Conner was now actually being invited for play dates for the first time since he was a toddler. Much more agreeable and thoughtful, his aggression was tremendously better. "We've come a long way from blind animal rage," his mother said. His teacher actually stopped me to ask what we'd done—she said he was like a different kid. His academic progress has been amazing, and the change in his ability to get along with the other kids has been like night and day."

Up to this point, Conner had never been formally diagnosed, though he'd been in special-ed classes for speech and reading problems for years. Eventually, the child was diagnosed with PDD-NOS, "with features of Asperger's syndrome." Michelle is glad they went through the formal evaluation process.

> *Though I already knew what the diagnosis was likely to be by the time we did it, getting that 'label' has made school officials much more willing to help accommodate him. Once teachers understood what was behind his outbursts, they got better at helping him avoid them, and his behavior improved. It's a feedback loop—so many of his behavior difficulties stem from feeling frustrated, and when he's less frustrated, he can behave more appropriately. I wish we'd gotten the diagnosis four years earlier.*

Peregrine Falcons are My Favorite Animals

The next interview with Conner took a rather surprising turn, though in hindsight it should have been clear all along. We had recently learned a new interviewing technique, and decided to explore Conner's attitude towards the animal kingdom. Conner was helpful:

> *My favorite animals are peregrine falcons, wolves, dogs, cats, and mongooses. Peregrine falcons are my*

very favorites. I just took a liking to them. I think falconry, hunting with falcons, is way cool. The falconer throws off the falcons with his hands to hunt for small prey like rabbits. One specific kind of falcon is the fastest animal on earth.

We found this new information most interesting, and were reminded that people needing medicines derived from birds tend to be thin-boned and wiry, just like Conner. We asked Conner to tell us more about birds: "Birds are different from any animal on earth. They are kind of prehistoric. Did you know what one of the first warm-blooded creatures on earth was a birdlike animal?"

We prescribed *Falcon* for Conner, a homeopathic medicine made from a drop of peregrine falcon blood. The main feeling of those needing *Falcon* is that of being restrained, confined, or trapped. Other symptoms of the medicine, in the homeopathic literature, include: anger when touched, violent anger, biting those around him, contrariness, discontentment, obstinacy, rage with swearing, and scratching others. A strong feature of children needing a homeopathic bird preparation is the desire, above all else, for freedom. The fact that Conner was engrossed in falcons and falconry was an additional confirmation for the prescription.

A Remarkable Response
We received a phone call from Michelle five weeks after Conner took the *Falcon* assuring us he was doing well. A month later, during our scheduled phone consultation, she bubbled:

Conner is doing fantastic! Better than ever. It's remarkable! He's solving problems with other kids rather than storming away, and is able to handle sit-

uations with his sister that never would have been possible before now. I would call him more resilient. It takes him five minutes to recover from an upset, rather than two hours. There has not been a single instance of Conner deliberately whacking me or his sister.

His academic improvement was amazing too; when we first gave the *Falcon* at the end of the school year, Conner was just beginning to read. Michelle described his progress: "Would you believe that Conner's reading tests at an eighth grade level, after having just learned to read last summer? He's been reading a 300 or 400-page book every week. Conner's even willing to try new foods and to engage in activities with people he doesn't know."

When we told Michelle what medicine Conner had received and why, she was fascinated; he had always shown an interest in raptors. She reiterated how much Conner hated being restrained. Even when he was quite young, if she tried to hold him tightly during a tantrum, "He would go ballistic, biting, screaming, and kicking. I know never to pin his arms."

Four months after first taking the *Falcon*, Conner was still progressing quite nicely. He had reached another stage of development, and no longer had any desire to sleep with his mom. Much more conscious of his body, Conner had developed a normal sense of modesty and a much more appropriate perception of social awareness and the normal rules of peer behavior. We asked Conner about his favorite animal again, to see if anything had changed. Again, he confirmed that it was a falcon.

They're cool, they're fast, and they're not a common favorite animal. It would be neat to be able to fly. You could hunt your prey and kill it and eat it extremely messily instead of having to use any manners. Carry it ruthlessly. Some falcons can die if they don't eat for three or four days.

Now, nineteen months after changing to *Falcon* and four years after beginning homeopathic care, all of the other positive changes have continued, and his sense of smell, keen as a toddler but missing entirely since age four, is back. Conner's reading is still way off the chart; this year he was placed in the Talented and Gifted program. During Conner's most recent appointment, Michelle glowed, "I'm thrilled. Conner is doing better than I could possibly have imagined. Now I have a kid that I can live with."

Not only has Connor continued to progress beautifully, but his mother has also benefited significantly from *Falcon*. Her chronic knee pain improved by 85%.

10

Monotones and Monologues
Parlez-Vous Aspie?

Although the severity and quality of their impairment
varies considerably, children along the autism continuum
universally struggle with communication. On the low-
functioning end of the spectrum, children often demonstrate delayed speech development. They may exhibit
limited language ability characterized by *echolalia*, or parroting of what they hear. On the high-functioning end of
the spectrum, children may demonstrate a precocious
vocabulary. Also common is an ability to read far beyond
their age level without truly understanding the meaning
of the words. They may sound like "little professors,"
talking over the heads of other children, and even some
adults, and rambling on about their special subject of
interest. Misunderstanding the social context of communication (*pragmatics*), children with ASD just don't get the
reciprocal give-and-take of NT conversation. During conversation, they frequently miss subtle inflection and
intonation, and are unable to grasp the intended meaning
of sarcasm, idioms, and polite expressions. Lacking
inflection, they may speak in a monotone, or stress sylla-
bles in an odd fashion.

Although the combination of a precocious vocabulary with minimal understanding of social context may be

endearing, even amusing, to adults, it poses serious difficulties for the child's social interactions with peers. She typically ends up confused, embarrassed, and alienated. Sadly, classmates who would never laugh at a child in a wheelchair can snicker or jeer mercilessly at an ASD kid's social *faux pas*. We have included two cases of children with semantic-pragmatic disorder (SPD) as examples of communication impairment typically seen on the high-functioning end of the spectrum. Though some consider SPD a distinct syndrome, in many ways it is very similar to AS, despite the increased language difficulties and better social skills.

Malik: Perseveration and Repetition to the Extreme

Malik, three and a half years old, was slow to walk, talk, and sit up. His mother, Jemila, noticed that he shook his hands and arms in a strange way when he became excited. Fearful and highly sensitive, he only wanted to be with mom, and refused to interact with anyone else. When others were around, Malik screamed in frustration, demanding 100% of Jemila's attention. His fussiness was unpredictable, and she never knew what was going to set him off. This created a definite strain on Jemila's social life since she could no longer get together with friends due to of the child's dependent nature. The stress on her became so great that the only way for her to cope was to avoid including the child in social situations. Jemila shared:

> *I always knew that Malik was behind developmentally, but it didn't worry me too much. Even though*

it was obvious that he had muscular and social development problems, I knew he wasn't dumb. Malik learned colors on his own, was able to recognize letters at two and a half, his attention span is fine, and he loves reading books.

But there were indications that everything was not quite on track. One of the moms in our carpool encouraged me to take Malik for testing. There were lots of things that Malik could not do by himself, or, at least, didn't think he could, like climbing up stairs or on a jungle gym. It's something with his muscles— they tighten up, and he yells for my help. Malik has a hard time climbing anything vertical. It's the same muscle tightening with bowel movements. Even if the stool is soft, getting it out is a major effort.

I have thought that Malik was autistic for quite a while. Rather than talking like other children his age, he repeats your questions. I'll ask him if he wants milk or juice, and he mimics the question back to me. It drives me up a wall. It was better for a while. He could actually answer me instead of merely looking dazed and repeating back whatever I said. Malik seems lost in his own world.

Watching anything spin is one of his favorite pastimes. Seeing objects in motion makes him jump up and down. I call it an involuntary muscle spasm. The great majority of the time, Malik walks on his toes. He can't feed himself. If he becomes really hungry, all hell breaks loose, and he loses all control of his muscles.

Malik is either very calm, or highly excitable and angry. During the calm moments, he enjoys reading books. At other times, he jumps up and down or loses his temper. If he gets messy when he eats, Malik freaks out and starts screaming.

Brushing his teeth turned into a screaming battle when he was one or two. Since he started attending a preschool co-op last year, the meltdowns have slowed down somewhat.

Mister Passion

According to his original school-district assessment, Malik was about a year behind his peers' development. The physical therapist identified a sensory processing disorder. Disinterested in engaging with other children, the youngster had not even interacted with his sister until he was three years old. The day that he did eventually connect with her was forever etched on Jemila's memory. Malik constantly remained by his mom's side like a puppy. He was fearful when his grandfather came to visit. Loud noises made him cry and scream. Being faced with crowded places like malls was an ordeal that inevitably ended with Malik grabbing onto Jemila for dear life.

I call him 'Mister Passion' because he's so full of extremes. He's gentle and kind one minute, like when he plays with animals. His touch is light, slow, and gentle. When he's calm, he's very calm. But, if you get him upset, he's a whole different kid. When Malik gets mad, watch out and duck your head; he throws whatever is around him. Like any child, he tests me to see what I'll do, but he reacts very intensely to scolding or reprimands. At school, Malik is very shy. In fact he didn't say one word to his preschool teacher all year! Malik simply doesn't talk there, but prefers to sit back and observe.

I use music a lot to calm Malik. He loves it and is terrific at keeping a beat. Maybe it comes from his dad, who is African and an avid musician. Once I

*left him with the babysitter for three hours. He was
at the keyboard when I left and when I returned!
Anything with buttons also fascinates him. And elec-
tricity. I catch him following the wires. Anything
that moves is likely to catch Malik's interest.*

Other than the stool problem, which was diagnosed
as encopresis, the child's only other physical complaint
was intermittent strabismus. Until the age of two, Malik's
eyes would cross so much that they would become stuck
in the middle.

Exceptional Features

 We found the tendency to muscular tightening
or spasms in the legs, bowels, and eyes to be odd
for a child this age. This is the first time we had
come across a child who, when overly hungry,
would "lose control of all of his muscles."

A number of Malik's other characteristics were not
so remarkable for a child on the autism spectrum: over-
sensitivity to noise, mood swings, social withdrawal,
developmental delays, toe walking, and perseveration.
The one other aspect of Malik that stood out was his physical appearance: he looked, in a way, like a little old man
rather than a small child. Malik's appearance, behavior,
and developmental delays led us to prescribe *Zincum*
(zinc). This medicine is also indicated for involuntary
muscle spasms, restlessness, and an adult-looking appearance. One year later, we changed the prescription, slightly, to *Zincum iodatum* due to the marked perseveration.

Some Amazing Changes

At his six-week appointment, Malik's mom mentioned
that a couple of old boils, which he had experienced earlier in his life, had erupted again shortly after taking the

medicine. Skin eruptions quickly following the ingestion of a homeopathic medicine are typically a good sign. Malik had begun talking to other people, was no longer bothered by crowded places, and just didn't get as mad or frustrated about life. Rather than throwing a tantrum, Malik was now able to appropriately say, "I feel upset." Screaming after naps had stopped. The week before, Jemila had been surprised when the boy climbed a jungle gym by himself without needing any help. Just one day earlier, he had scaled a vertical ladder at preschool, another first. The physical therapist noticed a sudden increase in confidence. The youngster had begun, for the first time, to sit down to breakfast and feed himself.

Jemila observed other positive changes. Malik was forming sentences more easily. Imaginative play came more spontaneously as well. His father commented that the youngster appeared to have made a developmental leap to play with more age-appropriate toys and act out stories with animation.

Some aspects had not yet changed: the spinning, muscle spasms, jumping up and down when excited, and noise sensitivity. Yet his overall change was impressive enough for Jemila to comment:

I'm just amazed at the big difference from when he started the remedy until today. My life is so much easier now from the changes that have taken place. You know, I was really at the end of my rope.

He's started to play with kids his age, which is wonderful progress. Before we came, he just had no interest in doing that. And Malik can play with his sister for much longer periods. His emotions can still be extreme, but he's learning to control them without needing to scream or cry. The biggest excitement for me is that he has continued to become more

social. Another improvement is that he definitely has
fewer spastic movements.

Malik was not stuck so often in repetitive activities
and the spinning had decreased. He was now climbing,
riding a tricycle, and his physical therapist told Jemila she
had never seen a child progress so quickly.

The steady improvement continued for a year after
beginning treatment. We gave Malik three doses of the
Zincum over the first four months, then switched to weekly doses, which his mother found more effective. Malik
was able to ask more logical, complex, and meaningful
questions. His behavior was still much more manageable,
and eye contact was more frequent. Stuttering was another problem helped considerably by the *zinc*. Eye to hand
coordination was also significantly better. Jemila
described the process:

> *It's as if a fog lifted from his brain. We find that*
> *Malik is more aware of our environment instead of*
> *being so absorbed in his own world. I see him get-*
> *ting more and more like a normal kid.*

We also recommended a gluten- and casein-free diet,
in the hope of easing Malik's bowel difficulties.

A Slight Adjustment in the Homeopathic Prescription
One year after we first saw Malik, he continued to
improve in most areas, though the encopresis was still
troublesome. Now that many of the other symptoms had
improved, the perseveration, though reduced, was the
most conspicuous complaint. Jemila explained,

> *It's driving me crazy! Malik talks about subjects*
> *obsessively, and I'm with him all day. He can go on*

and on for hours about batteries. 'Is that silver or gray? What's it for? What does it do?' 'Why isn't the light on?' I don't understand why he asks the same questions over and over when he already knows the answer. Then he gets upset if, out of exasperation, I don't answer.

Upon researching other zinc medicines, we discovered that *Zincum iodatum* (zinc iodide) was the only one listed in the homeopathic literature for "obsessive restlessness." It also covered the child's need to eat with great frequency. It is interesting, given the child's strong attraction to batteries, that some of them contain zinc. Shortly after starting the new medicine, Malik began inviting friends to his house. He was much better about letting Jemila talk on the phone without interruption. Another pleasant change was Malik's coming up to his mom, giving her a huge hug, and saying, "Sorry, mom" after he did something he shouldn't have. Malik was able to go comfortably for longer periods of time between meals. Jemila assured us, "I see a major leap every time I give him the medicine."

Jemila has added other therapies from time to time, such as Relationship Development Intervention (RDI), as time, money, and energy permit. She has found it extremely challenging to get the best overall care for Malik given her limited finances and her desire to also give adequate love and attention to his older sister, who is easily unnoticed and rarely asks for anything.

We have been treating Malik for three years. The transformation in the child is remarkable. At his last appointment Jemila beamed.

Malik is just doing so well. The way he can have conversations! Even his obsessions are much more on the level of typical kids. I no longer need to keep reminding, 'Now, Malik, you've asked me that already.' It's such a new thing that he is able to really take another person's perspective, which is quite a leap for an autistic child.

Noah: Vaccine and Antibiotic Damage

Noah, age five, was adept at calculating cube roots in his head. Prime numbers filled his brain, and he delighted in reciting series of numbers to himself while in the back seat of the car. This was a child who could multiply numbers in the millions in his head! Most children that age are barely adding or subtracting.

His precocious math skills weren't the only unusual thing about Noah. Though he seemed quite normal at times, neither his history nor his behavior was anything approximating average. During the pregnancy, Noah's father was unemployed, drowning his sorrows in alcohol. Enraged over the circumstances, Noah's mom, Diane, engaged in an ongoing battle with her husband. At six months of age, Noah developed a cold with a fever, for which he was treated with Amoxicillin. He subsequently vomited, and was found by his parents the following morning, floppy and unresponsive. Although he recovered at the hospital without obvious after-effects, the stage was set for later disability.

At birth, the newborn did not look at his mother. Crying incessantly, the baby was cross and grumpy, and eye contact was nearly nonexistent. Although the child's motor skills were mostly age-appropriate, Noah ambled awkwardly at eleven months, banging his head about a hundred times a day.

At seven months, Noah still adamantly refused to

look at anyone. At fifteen months, he suffered a high fever immediately after his MMR vaccine, another potential neurological insult. At eighteen months, while on a long car trip with his parents, the boy turned wild, yanking furiously on his mom's hair and gouging at her face. Over time Noah came to develop a hatred of adults and tried to attack any visitors to his home. The boy even lunged at one guest as she innocently blew up a balloon for him. By two and a half, his aggression was totally out of control. At three, Noah contracted chicken pox and the mumps, despite having received the MMR vaccination.

During this entire time, Noah did not speak a word, only making noises. Noah had absolutely no understanding of language. Thanks to his parents' diligent search for an explanation for their son's problems, he was finally diagnosed with Semantic Pragmatic Disorder (SPD), a language and communication disorder sometimes found in children with ASD. SPD is characterized by serious deficits in thought and language processing, poor social skills and behavior problems. It was not until his parents enrolled him in the 'Son-Rise' program, pioneered by Barry and Suzie Kauffman of the Options Institute, that Noah began to speak and develop more appropriately. The child began to read spontaneously, without any tutoring, revealing the intelligence that lay buried beneath his autistic features.

Solving the Cube Root of 729 in His Head

A European homeopath had treated Noah previously, but without any lasting success. When his parents brought him to our clinic, Noah exhibited "rigid moments", during which he clenched his muscles and chanted *"e-e-e-e"* with obvious distress. When his ears hurt on an airplane, Noah let out a loud and piercing *"a-a-a-a-a-h,"* to his father's and sister's embarrassment. Noah's overriding obsession with numbers and mathematics put off children his own age. Although Noah adored younger kids, he found relating to older children and adults difficult.

In emotional hyper-drive, if Noah accidentally scratched his head or knee he screamed bloody murder: "Cut my head off! Cut my leg off!" If ink dripped on his shirt, he ordered, "Cut that spot out!" An impulsive fellow, Noah had the habit of darting recklessly across the road in front of his house, explaining, "It's safer if you run too fast." The boy enjoyed pushing the envelope, trying to see how much he could push his way beyond the limits.

When we spoke with Noah alone, at first he was not easily engaged in conversation, then he curled up silently in the chair with an air of mild boredom. Simple questions gradually drew the boy out of his shell, but it was not until the subject of mathematics came up that Noah's spirit seemed to come alive. The boy proceeded, with steady concentration, shoulders hunched over and eyes eight inches from the desk, to scrawl numbers on a piece of paper. Quickly solving the cube root of 729, Noah demonstrated how he had multiplied nine three times and divided 729 by nine twice, all in his head. He then performed a few other math problems, one involving a negative number, as well as feats of multiplication that would challenge a nine- or ten-year-old. Impressive by any standard!

Noah's mom added that he preferred engaging with adults, who could give him knowledge. As long as the interaction was fact-based, it went fairly well. Unable to access genuine feelings, or to express himself spontaneously, Noah was unable to pay attention to subjects outside his circumscribed repertoire. We could not even stir up any enthusiasm for questions that kids we see in our practice normally find compelling, such as favorite foods, games, or toys.

Special Features

When considering a homeopathic medicine for Noah, a number of factors stood out. Noah was obviously intelligent, perhaps a savant. Despite his precocious knack for mathematics, Noah's interactive and social skills were poor, with little emotional depth. The youngster struck us as bright, but eccentric, and emotionally labile, with frequent episodes of aggression.

Since his mathematical abilities stood out as his most peculiar trait, our analysis of the case started there. It was obvious that Noah had a kind of mathematical fixation, in AS terminology, a "special interest." Able to perform calculations no five-year-old would be expected to do, he had no interest in talking about anything else. Noah had a rigid quality, with little ability to adapt to new situations, and a tendency to become fearful, distraught or aggressive if a situation was not to his liking. Though it was difficult to pin down exactly when he lost the capacity to learn and interpret language, it seemed possible that either the Amoxicillin or the MMR vaccine might have played a role in turning what would otherwise have been normal development in the direction of autism.

In prescribing for Noah, we were looking for a homeopathic medicine that was associated with difficulty in learning speech and language, rigidity, intense interests, lack of affection, and also had a connection with vaccine reactions.

Noah's case reminded us of two previous cases in our practice. One was a boy with OCD and Tic Disorder who counted obsessively and shared Noah's special aptitude for math. The second case was a child who had suddenly lost the ability to speak and become profoundly autistic following a febrile reaction to an MMR. Both of these boys had responded magnificently to *Silica*. Though their cases were not identical to Noah's, the similarities are evident; *Silica* covered the rest of Noah's symptoms as well. *Silica*, along with *Thuja* (Arbor vitae), is one of two medicines known in the homeopathic literature as specifics for post-vaccination symptoms. Though we usually do not prescribe by rote in this way, this keynote symptom did lend further confirmation to the use of *Silica* with Noah.

Mesorkavich Mesorkavich

Noah received a dose of *Silica*. The first week after taking medicine was uneventful, but by the first follow-up visit, he was showing considerable improvement. Much calmer, with much less crying and head banging, Noah was no longer having rigid spells or making chanting noises. His ability to attend to his daily Son-Rise program also improved markedly. Another significant change was an increase in Noah's imaginative play. Chattering on about his imaginary cat, Mesorkavich Mesorkavich (named after his old nanny), Noah recounted vivid tales of planes crashing into the cat's building (this was not long after the September 11th attacks). Noah's family of imaginary friends had grown, and his play was considerably more figurative and less literal. His self-expression was noticeably expanded as well, as evidenced by the increased menu of words he used to question or describe himself and the world around him. His mother, Diane, found the boy to be more reasonable overall.

Surprisingly, Noah had given up mathematics entirely for the time being. No longer occupied with cube roots and numbers, the youngster enjoyed playing normally with other children, who accepted him more easily. Noah's appetite increased and he stayed well throughout the winter months.

You Would Not Recognize Him!

Over the past two years, Noah has continued to do exceptionally well, needing only four doses of the *Silica*. During a recent visit, his parents described his progress:

Noah is improving so much. Recently, he began speaking about numbers again, but is now keen to include others in the discussions. My son is a lot more interactive. You simply would not recognize him! Language is age-appropriate, and Noah is very interested in having friends and relating to other people. We would say he chooses to be interactive 75% of the time; the rest of his time is devoted to his special interests. Echolalia is unheard of, and chanting rare. Noah's behavior and impulsivity have tapered to a manageable level. We've seen no head banging, except a little token striking on a cushion. Noah is now free of any muscle rigidity. He is still fascinated by the factors of 108, but shows little interest in cube roots.

At last report, Diane was overjoyed. "Noah's a different child." She recounted her son's great progress at school. Having transitioned to a mainstream classroom, to no one's surprise he was at the top of his class in math. The proud mathematician was still eager to display his math skills to anyone who showed an interest. Noah had made great strides in language development, and could speak in normal, coherent sentences. Echolalia, chanting, and head banging were completely eliminated. An avid student of piano, the youngster was learning to compose his own melodies. A computer aficionado, Noah was a quick study in setting up and configuring programs. He had retained his mathematical abilities in a healthy and balanced way, allowing him to open, naturally, to a wider range of interests.

Jimmy: A Human Calculator

Our child is a savant in math. Jimmy's eleven and he can tell you how many seconds there are in a month. But ask him what an ironing board is and he doesn't have a clue. The things he's interested in capture his awareness, but he's oblivious to the world around him. Jimmy was diagnosed with AS about two years ago. The only medication he takes is Concerta. His brother is also on the spectrum.

Maggie, Jimmy's mom, was a special-ed teacher and was overjoyed to tell us anything about her son that might provide a clue for us to help him. She had educated herself about homeopathy beforehand by devouring a couple of our books, and knew that anything unusual about pregnancy and labor might interest us.

All Jimmy Wants to Do is Draw Aircraft and Aliens

When Jimmy discovered a book of aircraft pictures, he simply couldn't put it down. We took him to an air show when he was two years old. Jimmy had gone down the rows and classified the planes: F-14, F-16, F-18, Stealth. He even corrected one of the pilots there. We thought it was adorable. This child was a walking encyclopedia of the artillery. He could recite all the specs. It never occurred to Jimmy that other kids couldn't care less about ammunition. He could easily entertain adults but couldn't talk to kids.

When we told Jimmy it was time to go to pre-school, he replied that he'd rather go back to bed. He hadn't the least interest in coloring or cutting out shapes. The teachers warned us at the time that he wasn't going to do well. They were dead on right. Jimmy's dad and I thought we had one smart little boy, but by October the school called us to say he wasn't making it at all. The special-ed teacher would tell him to do an assignment and, half an hour later, the kid wouldn't even have lifted a pen to begin. What they asked of him just didn't interest him so he wouldn't buy into it. Jimmy is very polite, very nice, so he's never rude or disrespectful like the other boys. He just doesn't do what they expect of the other children.

They pressured us to have Jimmy repeat kindergarten. He was the youngest boy in the class. Even when he repeated the year, he had difficulty. Here was the class all in a circle. And there was Jimmy. It's not that he lacks social skills. Jimmy has no problem finding someone to talk to, because he's just a really nice kid. He wants so badly to do well in school. Though he's only in fifth grade, Jimmy has tested at an eleventh-grade level in reading. He's gifted in math and his verbal ability is excellent. They actually put him on a TV show because listening to him is so entertaining.

It's an ordeal to get Jimmy up in the morning. Brushing his teeth, washing his face, putting on clean clothes—these are irrelevant to him. Drawing, reading, and playing computer games are how he would prefer to spend his day. Our boys have never had the opportunity to watch commercial TV, and they don't have Game Boys or Xboxes. So, Jimmy just draws. Even in his brother's books. Pictures of military gear, guns, aircraft, soldiers, aliens. As much as he loves to draw, he hates to write. The complaint from his teacher is that he doesn't do his work, but just draws.

A Polite, Sensitive, and Kind Child

One of the only three "polite" boys in his class, Jimmy would not consider acting rudely or disrespectfully. Popular with adults, Jimmy was an active participant in soccer, Cub Scouts, Math Olympiad, and a tech club. If he didn't want to do what was asked of him, he exercised a kind of passive resistance.

Jimmy's parents were particularly concerned about a period of sadness two months earlier that had "almost crippled him emotionally." They took it quite seriously, especially due to a history of depression on both sides of the family—his maternal grandparents and a paternal uncle who eventually committed suicide. The pediatrician agreed that Jimmy manifested all the classic signs of depression: nothing mattered to him, even food; he complained of feeling sad all the time; things he previously enjoyed no longer appealed to him; and he showed no interest in being around other kids. The school psychologist had warned Jimmy's parents that two years after children began taking Concerta or the other stimulants, they often experienced depression. The school nurse told them the same thing.

Maggie reported:

> *Out in your waiting room, Jimmy took it upon himself to read to the younger children. This is a kid who's tremendously sensitive and kind. Jimmy absorbs things. It affected him deeply when he saw the children drowning in Titanic. I just feel who the real Jimmy is hasn't been able to come out in a way that fits with his kindness and intelligence.*
>
> *Everybody likes Jimmy, but there's such a gap between who he really is and what he can do. They recruited him for the math team, but when there was an elite competition, they didn't invite him*

because of his lack of follow-through. Jimmy's a low-energy kid. His younger brother bounds into the day, but no matter how much energy Jimmy expends, he can't keep up. We were quite surprised he wanted to play soccer. He's a fast runner, but he never scores goals. Jimmy's just not pushed to do that. With the clarinet, it's deadly to get him to practice. All of our son's activities are limited by his energy.

Jimmy was prone to develop sores on his body, which he would inevitably make bigger by scratching. When younger, abnormally enlarged tonsils had been a problem for him. From age one to five, Jimmy was in and out of the emergency room every couple of months for ear infections and bad colds. An abnormally large, hairy mole appeared and kept growing larger and larger until it had finally been removed the previous fall.

During the last year, Jimmy had become very furtive, stealing candy, cookies, and food. Jimmy's dad even bought a lock box for the sweets to discourage the habit, but they still found the sandwiches he was sent for lunch hidden in his backpack. He would rather skip the main course and cut straight to the sugar.

A Whiz at Cube Roots of Pi and Armed Weapons
It was fascinating to speak with Jimmy personally:

I heard you gave my brother a very good medicine that helped him become more focused with his schoolwork, and I wanted to see if you could give me some, too. Something to help me be able to use my brain to its full potential. To figure out math problems in class more easily. I can get the problem done. I know what the answer is but I get a little off subject and then I completely forget the answer. I don't like that. Say I was talking to you about a math problem, then suddenly I went [the diplomas on the consulting room wall caught Jimmy's attention], "Wow, those are interesting medical degrees." I hate to play my clarinet. Getting my reed to work is hard. Say there's a note I have to make but I hear no sound coming out of the instrument. The problem is the idea of concentration. Or say I want to find what a word means in the dictionary but I can't seem to find it until the topic is already over. I need to be more direct and on the spot.

I like to do math in my head. Square roots, cube roots, fractions, pi. I know quite a few roots of pi [Jimmy recited them aloud.] The cube root of 27 is 3. The cube root of 2,197 is 13. I can get the problem in my brain in seconds, but I may not know how to explain it. 19,683 is the answer to 27 cubed. [We quickly checked Jimmy's answer and it was right on.] I would like to do other things like the clarinet but I'm not really motivated.

When we inquired about Jimmy's fascination with military gear and weapons, he explained,

I don't like violence or hurting anyone. That's the subject I've studied the most. My dad used to be a military pilot so we can talk about these things. You can ask me about any military weapon [here Jimmy rattled off a number of names which went right over our heads]. What's the most heavily armed tank in the world? I like to shoot a gun at targets but not at any animals. I would try to find the least violent alternative to stop violence.

We asked Jimmy to tell us what it felt like to be

depressed. He answered that nothing really seemed fun. That he would just sort of lie around and not do anything.

> *When I feel sad, I like rain. It's kind of like explaining rain. Or like trying to explain how to talk to a dumb person who can't speak. Or like trying to explain to somebody who's eight years old and about to die how to speak English. If it's rainy and gray outside, I just like it.*
>
> *I have a large and expanded vocabulary. Once I wrote a page of over one hundred words and their Latin roots. I can also read with almost complete fluency, including words that most of my peers would get stuck on.*

To prove his point, Jimmy picked up a homeopathic reference book from the desk and read from it quite accurately.

Though an exceptional public speaker, Jimmy had a distinct fear of standing out. In second grade, presenting math facts in front of the class made him very nervous. When the family went to a movie and his parents stayed to read the credits, Jimmy was mortified. "We have to get out of here," he would insist.

Exceptional Features

Jimmy's knowledge of weaponry was phenomenal. It is not uncommon for children with AS to develop a tremendous fund of knowledge, even a photographic memory, about a specific, often rather obscure subject, but a few other aspects of Jimmy stood out for us. First was his sincerity and motivation to get help, paired with his seeming disinterest in schoolwork. It was evident that he very much wanted help with concentration in order to accomplish his tasks with greater ease. Remember that he was the one who had asked his mother to bring him in for homeopathic treatment. This is not something we hear very often.

Secondly, this was an unusually polite child, particularly compared to some of the ruffians in his class. This was a politeness not merely born out of rigidity, but a sincere courteousness. Jimmy was exceptionally kind and considerate, and had a real desire to please. This nature, combined with the recurrent ear infections, limited stamina, and mathematical genius, led us to give Jimmy *Silica*. It is a mineral medicine for children and adults who are conscientious about doing well, but lack the grit and strength to carry out their intentions. We had used the same medicine successfully with a couple of other math savants, including Noah in the preceding case. Our previous experience led us to suggest to Jimmy's parents a possible secondary diagnosis of SPD.

Better and Better

Silica is known among homeopaths to be a medicine that can be slow to act, so we were willing to wait several months before drawing a conclusion as to whether it was the best medicine for him. At six weeks, his dad reported no dramatic change. Jimmy had developed a new interest in fabrics used for camping gear, his mission being to make the perfect jacket from a combination of Mylar and polypropylene.

At the three-month follow-up visit, Jimmy's parents were happy to report that he was getting straight Bs and was definitely more communicative and involved with people. A lady came up to Jimmy's mom and commented, "Your son is so engaged." When another boy fell into the lake at summer camp, Jimmy had demonstrated the presence of mind to plunge in with all of his clothes on and save him. Afterwards, when the counselor came up to thank him, Jimmy brushed it off, wanting no credit.

Another step forward, literally, was Jimmy and his dad's plan for a fifty-mile hike, a task that would have been far beyond Jimmy's previous level of physical capacity. Jimmy expounded on the pros and cons of internal versus external frame backpacks. He mentioned casually that he used to be afraid of other kids laughing at him, but wasn't anymore. We knew this was a good sign and a likely benefit of the *Silica.*

Jimmy needed a second dose of the medicine seven months later, after having eaten a Ricola cough drop, a menthol-containing product that can interrupt the action of homeopathic medicines. He did not relapse to anywhere near to the level he had presented at the first interview, but did become really tired after playing soccer, and felt like sleeping the second half of the school day. Jimmy explained why he believed that he needed a repetition of the medicine:

> *Grades are pretty important. They determine how your life will go. I want to get good grades, not bad grades, so I can feel good about myself. Now is the time to prepare for college. I'm feeling demoralized and much more tired. I want to get in the habit of getting better grades, not be left behind. Being held back would be the thing I definitely would not want to happen. I would feel really bad. I was held back in kindergarten. I didn't really care then, but I sure would now.*

Return visits are opportunities for us to get to know our patients more deeply. Once a child is doing well, we can relax and spend more time letting him say whatever comes into his mind. What he chooses to talk about and how he expresses himself confirm for us whether the medicine is correct and if he is progressing steadily. It's delightful for us to hear straight from the child himself that he is doing better. Jimmy obliged us.

> *I really don't like to stand out. It's one of those things you can't put a face to, you know. Maybe if you said something really crazy or dumb. Say you fell over in your chair. They wouldn't exactly be laughing at you, but they would think you were a strange, weird person.*

Self-consciousness is a prominent issue of *Silica*, which reassured us we had made a good choice. Jimmy went on:

> *I'd like more of that homeopathic stuff again. About seven or eight weeks ago, after I had that Ricola cough drop, I got more tired and it was harder to concentrate. Your medicine makes me more focused and less tired. It makes it easier to do school work. It makes everything a lot easier. The Concerta doesn't really seem to work. Explaining how it's supposed to work is like describing how a bird flies or how you walk. You just can't.*

We have been treating Jimmy for a year and a half. At his last visit, his mother proudly announced that the child's IQ had gone up twenty points from the last time he had been tested and that he had been accepted recently into the gifted program at school. Jimmy's teacher told his parents that, in his twenty-five-plus years of classroom experience, he had never seen a child make so much progress in one year.

PART THREE

Possible Causes of ASD and Questions about Diagnosis

11

Of Genes and Vaccines
Why So Many Children with ASD?

Current research indicates ASD has become an epidemic
and that the rates are rising. In 1999, the California
Department of Developmental Services (DDS) issued a
report indicating a 273% increase in autism rates
between 1987 and 1998.[19] Furthermore, from 1998 to
2002, the rates in California doubled; and in just one
year, from 2001 to 2002, there was an alarming 31%
increase.[20] Research has shown that over 81% of the
autism population in the California system was born after
1980.[21] The implications of this are staggering: autism is
on the rise, and we don't know why.

Although there is clearly an increase in prevalence,
researchers question whether the actual incidence of
ASD is on the rise, or if, due to greater *awareness* about
the condition, more children are being diagnosed.
Clinicians, teachers and parents are becoming increasingly well informed about the hallmark features of ASD, and
as a result, the number of diagnoses has simultaneously
increased. Additionally, changing diagnostic criteria,
varying research methodologies, and recognition of
autism as a spectrum of disorders may also have con-
tributed to a relative increase.

However, pediatric epidemiologist Dr. Robert S.
Byrd of the M.I.N.D. Institute of the University of

California at Davis, asserts that the increase in autism in California is a true increase and cannot be explained away by increased reporting and other artificial factors. Byrd acknowledges that speculation about the increase in autism in California has led some to try to explain it away as a statistical anomaly that has artificially inflated the numbers, but Byrd finds this speculation misguided at best.[22]

While the debate over a true or relative increase continues, all agree that the results of current epidemiological research on ASD are, without a doubt, startling. For now, we'll leave this question and take a direct look at the prevalence.

Just the Facts: How Common is ASD?

Epidemiological studies of prevalence mirror the overall trend demonstrated in California. Since 1979, the prevalence of ASD has nearly quadrupled. Below is a listing of some of these studies.

Year conducted	Prevalence of ASD, AS or PDD	Authors
1979	1 in 667 (ASD)	Wing & Gould [23]
1993	1 in 227 (AS)	Ehlers & Gillberg [24]
2001	1 in 159 (ASD)	Chakrabarti & Fombonne [25]
2002	1 in 175 (ASD)	Scott, Baron-Cohen, Bolton & Brayne [26]
2003	1 in 167 (PDD)	Fombonne [27]

The Genetics of ASD

Identifying the etiology (cause) of ASD has been a problem. Although many theories have been put forth, as of now, there is no clearly defined cause. As with most medical conditions where the etiology is elusive, most of the usual suspects are represented: genetics, environment, viral exposure, and trauma.

There is compelling evidence that genetics plays a role in ASD, though to what degree, researchers are uncertain. Genetic researchers frequently study twins to establish concordance rates, indicating how frequently both twins, identical or fraternal, share a specific condition. Shockingly, concordance studies have shown that 92% of identical twins (identical genetics) shared symptoms of ASD. With fraternal twins (whose genetics are not identical), the concordance rate drops to 10% for ASD.[28] Another study showed that there is a 3% chance that a sibling of an ASD child will have ASD himself.[29]

Of course, genes are only part of the story. If there is a true increase in ASD, it stands to reason that there would not be such a dramatic increase in prevalence of the disease in just two decades if genetics were the sole cause of ASD. Evolutionary biology simply doesn't work that fast! It takes 10,000 years or longer for a noticeable genetic shift to occur. Ultimately, these genetic studies suggest that there most probably are multiple genes, *in combination with* an environmental component, giving rise to ASD.

Possible Environmental Causes of ASD

Although there is a tremendous amount of speculation about numerous environmental causes, unfortunately, there is glaring lack of definite conclusions. It is challenging to scientifically demonstrate an environmental cause of ASD. First, the number of potential environmental causes runs into the thousands, and it has proven difficult to narrow the field. It is entirely possible that combinations of multiple environmental causes may interact to result in ASD. Secondly, even if we were able to narrow the field, it would obviously be unethical to conduct research that intentionally exposes an infant to the suspected environmental agent, so the best research can do is to use other research designs.

Vaccinations and Thimerosal: Is There a Link with Autism?

Until recently, vaccinations, including the measles, mumps and rubella (MMR), contained a mercury-based preservative called thimerosal. Many parents blame thimerosal for causing autism in their children. They assert that autism rates have exploded around the country in the past 15 years—the same period during which thimerosal became prevalent in vaccines. Since mercury is highly neurotoxic, some argue that early exposure may contribute to a child developing autism. In 2003, a study conducted by Geier & Geier based on the U.S. government's Vaccine Adverse Events Reporting System (VAERS) database found increases in the incidence of autism, mental retardation, and speech disorders following the administration of thimerosal-containing diphtheria, tetanus, and pertussis (DTaP) vaccinations as compared to thimerosal-free DTaP vaccines.[30]

The Food and Drug Administration (FDA), Centers for Disease Control (CDC) and the American Academy of Pediatrics (AAP), however, argue that thimerosal and vaccinations are safe and have strongly criticized Geier & Geier's 2003 study. In spite of their confidence that no link exists, as a precautionary measure, the AAP and CDC issued a joint statement instructing vaccine manufacturers to reduce or eliminate thimerosal in vaccines.[31]

In our clinical experience, while the majority of our ASD patients do not overtly exhibit negative results from their immunizations, some seem to have suffered such devastating effects as profound speech delay, social withdrawal, mutism, and psychoneuromotor abnormalities. The proximity of these symptoms to the time of having received one or more immunizations, while not definitively causative, is too conspicuous to ignore (See Paolo's case in chapter eight).

Viruses, Trauma and Toxins

One environmental theory of ASD involves prenatal exposure to viral or other infections. Those implicated include herpes, rubella, rubeola, varicella, toxoplasmosis, and syphilis. However, these are mainly single cases, and there is not yet enough evidence to validate these theories.[32] [33] [34]

The available research is inconsistent on whether prenatal or birth trauma such as the use of forceps or suction during delivery is associated with autism. The data provides only marginal support for the association of birth trauma with low-functioning autism, and the association with High-Functioning Autism (HFA) is even less convincing.[35]

Teratogens, or fetus-damaging chemicals, have also been studied. There is strong evidence suggesting an association between autism and thalidomide; and an animal studies link has been demonstrated with the drug Depakote (valproic acid.)[36] Also, drug use, including cocaine, during pregnancy was associated with an 11% increase in autism, and 94% of those exposed to drugs demonstrated a delay in language.[37]

Speculation and Treatment

For now, we can only speculate as to what causes ASD. Genetics plays a role, and most likely, environmental causative factors are involved as well. Hopefully, we will have more definitive answers to these questions over the next decade. For us, as clinicians treating children with ASD, speculating on the potential cause takes a back seat to focusing on the challenges and limitations the patient with ASD is facing right now, and how we can help.

12

Alphabet Soup
Diagnoses That Accompany or Disguise ASD

More often than not, children with ASD don't fall neatly into one diagnostic category. In fact, up to two-thirds of children with ASD have additional (coexisting) psychiatric labels.[38] These additional diagnoses read like an alphabet soup: ADHD, ODD, ADD, OCD, SID, TS, LD, NLD, CAPD, and others (see Glossary). As the nature of ASD is multi-dimensional, it is sometimes difficult to tease apart these accompanying diagnoses.

In light of this complexity, it shouldn't be surprising that misdiagnosis is common. Because ASD shares many characteristics and symptoms with these other diagnoses, it is very common for kids with ASD to be misdiagnosed with another condition before receiving the correct (or additional) diagnosis of ASD. For example, what can appear on the surface as anxiety, depression, or ADHD may actually at its core be ASD. With any form of treatment, the goal is to treat the root of the problem and a mistaken diagnosis may lead to improper, or ineffective, treatment of what is, in fact, ASD.

ADHD and ASD
We have treated more than 3,500 children with ADHD and ADD. Over the last few years, we've cultivated more sophisticated radar for ASD. And now, looking back on

many of those ADHD and ADD children, we realize that the diagnosis of ASD would have been a better fit. According to OASIS, an online resource that conducts informal surveys of parents of AS children, 65% of children who had initially been described as ADHD latter received a diagnosis of AS. Additionally, 44% of parents stated that their child had been given a dual diagnosis of AS and ADHD.[39]

Without an understanding of the root cause, it is easy to see how the symptom picture of ADHD can overlap with that of ASD. Kids with ADHD lack *social control.* Within the school setting, their impulsivity, hyperactivity and inattention often land them in the principal's office. By contrast, kids with ASD may also find themselves in the principal's office, but the root issue is a lack of *social understanding* rather than social control. Thus, although the behaviors, and the unwanted consequences, may be the same, the underlying issue is very different for each child. For example, consider Brook.

Playing with other children did not come easily to Brook. All too often his hyperactivity and impulsiveness would spiral out of control during group activities, quickly overwhelming his peers. He liked to be in control when playing with others, and despite frequent protests from his playmates, he would bark orders at them. Rigid and dictatorial, Brook allowed his peers very little improvisation or spontaneous play. It was his way or the highway. He would come down hard on kids who broke rank, and the other children in his class were beginning to avoid him during play times. Could Brook have ADHD? ASD? Or both?

For different reasons, children with ADHD and ASD often find reciprocal play difficult. The give and take of playing a game involves being receptive to a playmate's suggestions and ideas. Impulsive and lacking social control, a child with ADHD may be unable to censor his behavior. Lacking restraint, kids with ADHD can quickly turn an enjoyable game into complete chaos for everyone, alienating their playmates in the process. Kids with ASD, in contrast, generally feel safer with routine and predictable outcomes. Sticking doggedly to routine, a child with ASD may resort to ruling with an iron fist. Lacking the social understanding and communication skills required to remain open to another kid's ideas, a child with ASD can appear dictatorial. They are determined to be right, because being wrong implies an unpredicted, and unwanted, outcome.

Depression and ASD

Children and adolescents with ASD are prone to developing mood disorders such as depression. Since socializing doesn't come easily, they find it challenging to fully connect with their peers. Particularly as they enter junior high school, they tend to feel isolated and on the fringe. Since the give and take of a reciprocal relationship does not happen naturally for them, friendships are frequently elusive.

Adolescence is a challenging and confusing time for nearly everyone. For teens with ASD, the fears about not fitting in, or being "different," are magnified many times. A University of Michigan study indicated that over half of the participants with ASD age 13 and older had a diagnosis of depression.[40]

Anxiety and ASD

Given the inconsistencies and unpredictability that exists in the world, it should come as no surprise then that many kids with ASD suffer from anxiety. In fact, up to 74% of people with ASD experience anxiety and fears.[41] For youngsters who rely on routine and structure to cope with the anxiety and fear, being thrown into a new and chaotic world of noisy school children, for example, could be paralyzing. Adhering rigidly to routine may serve to keep the anxiety at bay.

Obsessive-Compulsive Disorder (OCD) and ASD

Children with ASD typically engage in their special interests with extreme single-mindedness. These ritualistic and repetitive behaviors are sometimes confused with the obsessive thoughts and compulsions associated with OCD. The qualitative difference between the two disorders lies in how the youngster *experiences* the obsession. With ASD, engaging in the special interest is pleasurable and often relaxing. In fact, a child with ASD may engage his grand passion in order to calm himself, and the amount of time spent with the special interest can be a good barometer for parents of their child's stress level. By contrast, the obsessive thoughts of individuals with OCD are experienced as unwanted and tormenting. In other words, these thoughts are experienced as increasing rather than reducing stress. It is easy to see how a misdiagnosis of OCD can occur. On the surface, a grand passion may present as OCD compulsivity. Just underneath the surface, however, may be the proper diagnosis of ASD.

Tics, Tourette Syndrome (TS), and ASD

Tic disorders, including TS, can involve involuntary movements that are repetitive in nature. These may be simple or complex movements of the body such as grimacing, blinking, throat clearing, and involuntary vocalizations. Tic disorders should not be confused with "self-stimming" behaviors, often associated with ASD, which are also repetitive in nature.

In a Swedish population study of individuals with

AS, 20% met full criteria for TS, and a full 80% had tics of one kind or another.[42]

Oppositional-Defiant Disorder (ODD) and ASD

Children with ODD tend toward hot heads and fiery tempers. They hate to be told what to do—by anyone. These kids can make the pleasantries of daily life a thing of the past. At worst, parents are afraid to open their mouths for fear the child will jump down their throats. Any question, remark, or request can turn into a major fight. These children may continue to tantrum well into the age where they should be developing maturity and self-control. An oppositional child can push their parents, family, teachers, and everyone else in the vicinity to the limit of their patience, peace, and sanity.

Children with ASD can also behave in an oppositional manner, but again, the underlying root cause for this behavior may be very different. For instance, Robbie had been engrossed by model train engines since age seven, and his basement was crisscrossed by a web of train tracks. Chief engineer Robbie easily became single-mindedly obsessed when passing a shop containing locomotives. If anyone made the mistake of coming between Robbie and his trains, he didn't take it lying down. Even when the store was about to close, with lights going off, floors being swept and mopped, Robbie would plant himself squarely in the train aisle, oblivious to the clerk's blatant reminders. On more than one occasion, his parents had carried him, kicking, spitting, and screaming from toy stores. Attempting to reason with the young chief engineer was to no avail. Nor did setting time limits ever seem to work. A quick trip to the mall could take an extra hour if the boy caught sight of a store that sold trains. If on a tight schedule, Robbie's parents were exceedingly careful to avoid such shops, navigating a circuitous route through the mall, doubling back and ascending and descending multiple escalators in order to do their shopping.

While on hearing this information, a professional unfamiliar with ASD might misdiagnose Robbie with ODD, a knowledgeable professional would quickly see his core issues are ASD related. Obsessive fascination with special interests is commonly at the root of temper tantrums and extreme defiance, especially when those special interests are interrupted. Often, when kids with ASD are in the middle of a routine, they need to see it through to completion. Like their cherished trains, they too may only be able to operate on one track at a time.

Sensory Integration Dysfunction (SID) and ASD

During an interview with Temple Grandin, noted autism researcher Tony Attwood inquired, "If you had ten million for research, how would you spend the money?" Grandin replied, "One of the areas I would spend it on is figuring out what causes all the sensory problems.... It's something that makes it extremely difficult for persons with autism to function."[43]

Many children with ASD share Ms. Grandin's struggle with sensory integration, and their sensitivities can greatly interfere with their daily routine. A child can be either over- or under-responsive to sensory stimuli such as touch, taste, sound or scent. A child with ASD who is over-responsive may develop sensory defensiveness, avoiding sounds, tastes, textures, touch and smells that an NT wouldn't give a second thought. A child who is under-responsive may seek more intense sensations or sensory experiences of an extended duration.

Although not listed as one of the core diagnostic criteria of AS in the DSM-IV, sensory problems can have a negative impact on the child's capacity to learn, to function in socially appropriate ways, and to perform everyday tasks of living.

Addressing the Root Cause

It is not uncommon for ASD to masquerade as other conditions. What appears on the surface, may, in fact, not be the correct diagnosis, or is one of two or more diagnoses. Either way, when it comes to treatment of children with ASD, it is important to look beyond the superficial behaviors in order to address the root issues. Treating superficial behaviors without addressing the real problem is just a patch-up job that rarely holds. As homeopaths, it is this underlying imbalance we attempt to understand and address.

13

Naming the Problem
The Challenges and Benefits of Diagnosis

Although official diagnoses like those listed in the DSM-IV may sound definitive and final, in reality they are often questioned and debated. The diagnosis of AS is no exception. Children are unique individuals who, thankfully, don't always fall neatly into diagnostic boxes. There are currently no definitive diagnostic lab tests for AS, and as a result, diagnosis is based on a developmental history and observed behavior. Developing criteria that distinguish AS from other diagnoses is an ongoing process.

Will the True Diagnosis Please Step Forward!
Here is a fictitious case that illustrates the difficulties of diagnosing AS: The Johnsons took their son, Sam, to his pediatrician for an assessment. Since infancy, there had been something different about the youngster. He rarely made eye contact, hated hugs, and became irate whenever something interrupted his routine. Now that he was entering third grade, his parents had become aware of how awkwardly he interacted with his classmates. Though his IQ was above average, and his vocabulary impressive, he remained friendless and on the social fringe.

The pediatrician assessed Sam, and after asking some questions and thinking back over her past visits with Sam, began to suspect that Sam had high-functioning autism (HFA) with a dual diagnosis of ADHD. After explaining what she knew about HFA, she referred Sam to a clinical child psychologist for testing. The Johnson family left her office feeling relieved to have a diagnosis, but also confused. Sam didn't seemed much like the children with autism they had met. They knew something about ADHD, but they were not familiar with the term HFA. They immediately made an appointment with the psychologist, anxious to learn more about their son and his condition.

Following a psychological assessment, the child psychologist told the Johnsons that their son showed all of the typical developmental and behavioral signs of AS. Testing results also indicated a diagnosis of AS. "But," the Johnsons questioned, "Sam's pediatrician had suspected high-functioning autism and ADHD. Is it possible that he has just ADHD or HFA rather than AS? We're confused about all these different diagnoses and how much they seem to overlap! Is it really that important that we label him at all? How will having a diagnosis like this affect him?" The psychologist took time to answer each of their questions. She explained each diagnosis, reassuring them that it wasn't uncommon for different clinicians to come up with different diagnoses, especially within the realm of developmental disabilities. She concluded by saying that it was important that Sam have the appropriate diagnosis.

Many parents such as Sam's report to us that their children received different diagnoses from different clinicians—all well-trained, knowledgeable professionals. Many parents express feelings of frustration and bewilderment when they find themselves in this situation. And some may question the utility of having their child diagnosed in the first place. Though the process of obtaining a diagnosis and then discussing it with your child may, at times, feel frustrating, painful or confusing, ultimately, it will benefit your child.

How is Diagnosis Beneficial?

What is really gained by formal diagnosis, and how is having a diagnostic foothold advantageous? Additionally, what are some of the concerns commonly raised by parents regarding the issue of diagnosis?

During an interview between Tony Attwood and Temple Grandin, Tony asked Temple how her parents presented her diagnosis to her. She replied,

> *Actually, I was kind of relieved to find out there was something wrong with me. It explained why I wasn't getting along with the other kids at school and why I didn't understand some of the things teenagers did, like when my roommate would swoon over the Beatles. She'd roll around on the floor squealing in front of the* Ed Sullivan Show. *I'd think, yeah, Ringo is cute, but I wouldn't roll around on the floor...*[44]

For many parents of ASD children, as well as adults diagnosed with ASD, it is deeply relieving to have a diagnostic explanation to confirm one's personal experience. Years of confusion and wondering "what's happening here?" are finally replaced with an explanation. It can be of immeasurable assistance in aiding parents, children and providers to understand why a kid is having so much difficulty in school and with her peers. Interestingly, an informal survey conducted by the OASIS group (Online Asperger Syndrome Information and Support) indicated that nearly all of the adults with AS confirmed that they would have liked to known about their diagnoses earlier.

Unanimously, they recommend that parents share the diagnosis with their children.[45]

It is understandable that some parents may feel reluctant to seek the proper diagnosis for their child, or may think that a diagnosis doesn't matter. However, the pros of diagnosis generally outweigh the cons. A proper diagnosis serves to orient parents so that they know where to look for accurate information about effective interventions, therapies, treatments, insurance reimbursement, and educational assistance. Diagnosis empowers parents and children with knowledge that can make a positive impact on a child's life. Thus, as family physicians, we encourage parents to obtain a proper diagnosis and gain access to the many services available to benefit their child.

Concerns About Receiving a Diagnosis

Sometimes parents feel very uncomfortable labeling kids with psychiatric diagnoses. They argue that labeling a child does more harm than good. In a medical climate where the tendency is to give a diagnosis for every deviation from the norm, this sentiment is understandable. When we attach a label to a child, the label can create a tendency to lose sight of her uniqueness and individuality. Sometimes parents fear that their child will be perceived as disabled, and be discriminated against or no longer treated as an individual. In addition, a child diagnosed with any behavioral issue risks being stigmatized by her peers. Socially, especially during the middle school years, kids often fear differences. Thus, the label of AS, or any label for that matter, may further marginalize children who are already alienated from their peers.

Although the diagnostic process can be distressing to parents and kids alike, it's essential to keep in mind that *a child with AS is much more than any label will ever tell!*

It's also extremely important that you let your child know that. A child with AS has multiple strengths and weaknesses, just as any child does. Parents should not lose sight of the big picture, the complex process of their wonderful, unique child developing into a wonderful, unique adult.

All of these concerns about how a child will respond to diagnosis are valid, and how and when a diagnosis is conveyed to the child can make a big difference in how the information is received. Many parents dwell on what and when to tell their AS child. You are certainly not alone, even though you may feel that way. Fortunately, there are numerous resources that provide guidance in this arena.

Explaining the Diagnosis

Tony Attwood, one of the most prominent clinicians working in the field today, likens AS to having a brain that's "wired differently, not defectively." This insight speaks volumes. Simon Baron-Cohen, a researcher from the University of Cambridge, suggests that conceiving of AS as a "different cognitive style as opposed to a deficiency" may seem subtle and unimportant, but in fact, could make a substantial impact on how the family and child integrate the diagnosis.[46] Baron-Cohen argues that this shift could mean the difference between whether the diagnosis is received as a family tragedy such as schizophrenia, or whether it is akin to being told that the child has some unique feature such as being left-handed or having perfect pitch.

Certainly, comparing left-handedness to AS understates the challenges faced by those with AS, but Baron-Cohen's hyperbolic point is well taken. There is a wide range of "normal," and differing from the somewhat arbitrary norms of society need not take on a negative nuance. Additionally, depending on the situation and context, a different cognitive style may be immensely advantageous. Hans Asperger himself emphasized how valuable people with AS are to society;[47] contributing ideas, professional skills, and talents that benefit society as a whole.

Homeopathy: Looking Beyond Diagnosis to Valuing Brains Wired Differently

So where does homeopathy fit in to the question of diagnosis? Although diagnosis certainly has its advantages, as mentioned above, from a homeopathic perspective, a diagnosis mainly serves as a starting point. More specifically, homeopaths treat people *with* diagnoses. As William Osler, the father of modern medicine, wrote, "Ask not what disease the person has, but what person the disease has."[48] This is where homeopathy shines! The characteristics listed as the diagnostic criteria for AS are only a beginning for determining exactly which homeopathic medicine will be of most benefit to the individual child.

PART FOUR

What Else Can You Do to Help Your Child with ASD?

14

Other Alternative
Treatments Worth
Considering

If you are the parent of an ASD child, you have probably combed bookstores and the Internet looking for *anything* that might help your child. Fortunately, many resources are available, both conventional and alternative (see Appendix). Dietary approaches, for example, are very common for the treatment of ASD. In some cases, homeopathy is so successful that dietary modifications are unnecessary. But, with other children, the most rapid and impressive results come from combining homeopathy with dietary changes or supplements. Most dietary approaches are compatible with homeopathic treatment, particularly the elimination diets, nutritional supplementation, and Nambudirapad Allergy Elimination Technique (NAET).

Approaches such as mercury detoxification using chelating agents seem a bit invasive to a homeopath, given the gentleness of our medicines, but we do acknowledge they have been quite useful in helping some youngsters, and we are willing to try working with practitioners and patients who are using chelation therapy.

Diets

Two well-known diets showing promise for the treatment of ASD are the gluten-free/casein-free diet (GF/CF) and the Specific Carbohydrate Diet (SCD™). These two approaches are probably familiar to most savvy parents of children on the autism spectrum, but for those new to dietary treatment of autism, a brief review of the main concepts of each diet may be useful. Some parents may also not be aware of the Feingold Program (FP), which eliminates additives, preservatives, colorings, salicylates and other factors that may affect children's health and behavior. In use with behaviorally challenged kids for over thirty years, the FP was initially controversial, but is now fairly widely accepted and clinically shown to be beneficial in many cases.

Leaky-Gut Syndrome

Each of these nutritional approaches is based on the underlying concept that various food substances, their derivatives, or the toxins and byproducts of bacterial, viral or fungal metabolism can inflame and damage the lining of the intestine (mucosa), making it more permeable. This allows those substances to be absorbed into the bloodstream and to possibly cross the protective blood-brain barrier, causing neurological and behavioral symptoms. The notion that some children have increased intestinal permeability is at the root of many of these theories of dietary elimination and management, and this seems to be supported by a wide range of research.[49]

Inflammation and damage to the mucosa may be caused by a variety of agents and processes. Gluten and casein, yeast overgrowth, bacterial toxins, viral infections such as measles, reduction in phenol sulfur transferase (which protects against leaky-gut syndrome), and damage from heavy metals such as mercury, lead, arsenic, cadmium, and antimony may all play a role in the development of leaky-gut syndrome.

The "leaky-gut" refers to the spaces created between the cells of the intestinal lining. These spaces can act, paradoxically, both as a sieve through which toxins and byproducts pass easily, and as a barrier to nutrient absorption. These two problems can lead to malnutrition, digestive difficulties (which are often seen with ASD), and bacterial and fungal overgrowth. When fewer nutrients are absorbed, a supportive environment develops for the growth of pathologic bacteria and yeast (this process is called *dysbiosis*) in both the small and large intestines. The increased bacterial and fungal load creates more toxic byproducts, which leak out of the small intestine into the bloodstream. This increases demands on liver function, and ultimately, may be implicated in the neurological and behavioral effects associated with ASD.

A 1996 study found that 43% of a group of 21 autistic children with no previously diagnosed intestinal disorders had leaky-gut syndrome, while no evidence of leaky gut was found in the (non-autistic) control group.[50] Horvath and Perman, in a 2002 review of the literature confirmed this idea finding:

> *Recent clinical studies have revealed a high prevalence of gastrointestinal symptoms, inflammation, and dysfunction in children with autism. Mild to moderate degrees of inflammation were found in both the upper and lower intestinal tract. In addition, decreased sulfation capacity of the liver, pathologic intestinal permeability, increased secretory response to intravenous secretin injection, and decreased digestive enzyme activities were reported in many children with autism. Treatment of digestive problems appears to have positive effects on autistic behavior.[51]*

The Gluten-Free/Casein-Free Diet (GF/CF)

In the last few years the GF/CF diet has become a mainstay in the treatment of ASD. Since the early 1980s, research has been accumulating to suggest that at least part of the mystery of autism has to do with the leakage of peptides (short chains of amino acids broken down from proteins) from a leaky gut into the blood stream. These peptides have endorphin-like (pain-relieving and pleasure-inducing) effects. When peptides cross the blood-brain barrier, they can alter neurotransmitters and may impact brain development or trigger some of the behavioral characteristics of autism.

Researchers including Dr. Karl Reichelt of Norway, Dr. Paul Shattock of the U.K., and Dr. Robert Cade in the U.S. have done research on the peptides (called opioids) in the urine of people with autism and found them to be the result of the incomplete breakdown of gluten from proteins in cereal grains (wheat, rye, barley, and oats) and casein from proteins in milk products.[52] The peptides gliadomorphin (from gluten) and casomorphin (from casein) chemically resemble morphine, and may be associated with opiate-like symptoms in the body, including painlessness, self-stimulatory or self-injurious behaviors, and disorientation.

Peptides with opioid activity derived from dietary sources, in particular, foods that contain gluten and casein, pass through an abnormally permeable intestinal membrane and enter the central nervous system (CNS) to exert an effect on neurotransmission, as well as producing other physiologically-based symptoms. Numerous parents and professionals worldwide have found that removal of these exogenously derived compounds through exclusion diets can produce some amelioration in autistic and related behaviors.[53]

Removing gluten and casein from the diet has produced considerable benefit in many children and adults with ASD. The earlier in the autistic child's life the elimination diet is begun, the more profound its effects seem to be, because gluten- and casein-derived opioids affect brain development. Some children have responded so favorably to the diet that they are no longer considered autistic, while others experience partial improvement in symptoms. Certain children are more susceptible to gluten (as in celiac disease), and some more to casein, but it is advisable to remove both completely from the diet. (See sidebar.)

Recent research on oats indicates that, at least for celiac disease (gluten intolerance), in adults, and perhaps in children as well, oats may be permissible in moderation. No research has been done on ASD in this regard.[54]

Foods to Avoid on the GF/CF Diet

Foods Containing Gluten
• all foods containing wheat, barley, rye, oats, or their derivatives
• wheat, whole-meal, whole-wheat, and wheat-meal flours, wheat bran, semolina
• barley, barley malt, barley-based drinks, barley fruit drinks, malted drinks, beer
• rolled oats, oatmeal, oat flour
• rye products, including flour and bread
• kamut, amaranth, spelt
• bread, cereals, pasta, or noodles made from any of the above grains.
• muesli yogurt
• bread pudding, pastry, pies, cookies, or other baked goods made from the above grains

- some pepper compounds
- shoyu (made with wheat)
- ready-mix spices
- some seasoning powders
- certain brands of mustard
- certain medicines

Foods Containing Casein
- all dairy products from the cow and goat including milk, cheese, butter, ice cream, buttermilk, cottage cheese, cream cheese, yogurt, and frozen yogurt.
- all products that contain casein, hydrolyzed casein, lactic casein, or caseinates
- some diet drinks and supplements
- some beverages
- hydrolyzed proteins
- coffee whiteners
- infant formulas
- pharmaceutical products

Many products contain hidden casein. Be sure to read the labels of any processed or packaged food or pharmaceutical product. If in doubt, contact the manufacturer for detailed information.

It is useful to give autistic children at least a three- to six-month trial on the GF/CF diet to see if autistic symptoms abate or disappear. Those who respond should stay on the diet at least a year, but many benefit from following it indefinitely. Symptoms may reappear when gluten and casein are reintroduced, even in small amounts. (See Appendix for resources on GF/CF diets.)

The Specific Carbohydrate Diet (SCD™)

This elimination diet goes a few steps further than the GF/CF diet, and for those ASD children who do not respond to GF/CF after a three- to six-month trial, it may provide an effective alternative.

The SCD™ was developed in 1951 by Sydney Valentine Haas, MD, for treating celiac disease, an inability to digest gluten. Dr. Haas' work has been carried on by biochemist Elaine Gottshall, M.Sc.. Her book *Breaking the Vicious Cycle* has been an inspiration to thousands of people with irritable bowel disease, Crohn's disease, ulcerative colitis, and more recently, many parents of children with ASD, who have reported remarkable results.

The SCD™ is based on a Paleolithic diet of foods that break down into single, easily absorbed molecules. The SCD™ eliminates complex sugars, starches and chemical additives in order to starve the yeast and bacteria in the gut that thrive on them. Following the diet for a year allows the intestinal tract to heal, although in many cases, results are often obtained much sooner. In the beginning of treatment, the die-off of microorganisms can cause increased symptoms for a few weeks; this is considered by SCD™ proponents to be a good sign. According to the SCD™ website:

> *The Specific Carbohydrate Diet™ is biologically correct because it is species appropriate. The allowed foods are mainly those that early man ate before agriculture began. The diet we evolved to eat over millions of years was predominantly one of meat, fish, eggs, vegetables, nuts, low-sugar fruits. Our modern diet including starches, grains, pasta,*

legumes, and breads has only been consumed for a mere 10,000 years. In the last hundred years the increase in complex sugars and chemical additives in the diet has led to a huge increase in health problems ranging from severe bowel disorders to obesity and brain function disorders. We have not adapted to eat this modern diet as there has not been enough time for natural selection to operate. It therefore makes sense to eat the diet we evolved with.[55]

SCD™ Generally Not Allowed and Allowed Foods

Not Allowed
- grains (rice, wheat, corn, oats, etc.)
- processed foods
- starchy vegetables (potatoes, yams, etc.)
- canned vegetables of any kind
- flour
- processed meats
- sugar, no sweeteners other than honey and saccharin
- milk products except for specially prepared homemade yogurt fermented for 24 hours.
- yeast
- tofu and most soy products

Allowed
- meats
- fish
- eggs
- unprocessed cheese
- butter
- vegetable oils

- beans, miso, tamari (after three months)
- fresh vegetables
- fresh fruits or fruits canned in their own juice
- nuts
- seeds (after three months)
- artichokes
- avocados
- honey
- spices (not spice mixtures, which often contain grains)

Though such a diet may seem too restrictive for some, it is apparently a godsend to those with few other options. For those interested in trying the SCD™ diet for ASD, see the Appendix for more resources.

The Feingold Program

Based on the elimination of harmful additives, colorings, preservatives and aspirin-like compounds called salicylates, the Feingold Program was originated by Dr. Benjamin Feingold, an allergist and pediatrician at Kaiser-Permanente Hospital in San Francisco. Feingold had observed a relationship between certain food additives, salicylates and behavior, especially in children with ADHD. Quite controversial when originally proposed in the late '70s and early '80s, the Feingold Program has stood the test of time, helping thousands of children decrease their food sensitivities, hyperactivity, ASD, and behavior and learning problems.

Most of the early research on the Feingold Diet was mixed. As an example, one 1981 study that tested children already on the Feingold diet based on their reaction to food coloring showed no difference between the food coloring group and controls.[56] Another study from Spain in the same early-'80s time frame was more positive. Of children who showed allergy-like symptoms, but for whom no allergies were found after extensive testing, 58% showed reaction to dyes, 34% reacted to benzoates, and 8% to salicylates.

Two more favorable studies based on the Feingold Diet were conducted in Australia by K.S. Rowe. In the first study, 72% of subjects improved on a six-week trial of the Feingold Diet, and 47% remained improved even after liberalization of the diet three to six months later.[57] In a later study, Rowe found that "behavioral changes in irritability, restlessness, and sleep disturbance are associated with the ingestion of tartrazine (a yellow food coloring) in some children."[58]

Despite the mixed results of research studies, anecdotal reports of the effectiveness of the Feingold Program in reducing symptoms in children with ADHD and ASD have been quite impressive. From the Feingold Program website: "Many families have reported that symptoms of autism spectrum disorders are reduced by using Stage One alone, or a combination of Stage One and a gluten-free, casein-free diet."[59]

A survey by the Autism Research Institute indicated that:

> ...the diet with the biggest success rate was the Candida Diet (52%), followed by the Feingold Diet (50%). 45% of the children improved with the removal of dairy (casein), and 41% improved with the removal of wheat (gluten). Removal of both gluten and casein together was not addressed in this survey.[60]

The Feingold Association of the United States (FAUS)

provides members with a comprehensive "food list" of brand name foods and household products that are free of the prohibited additives. A members-only online "bulletin board" is also an invaluable source of support, recipes, and ideas for many Feingold parents. For parents of ASD children who are looking for a dietary approach that can have considerable effect, either alone or in combination with the SCD™ or GF/CF diet, the two-stage Feingold Program is certainly worth checking out.

The Feingold Program[61]

Stage One
During Stage One the following items are eliminated:

- Artificial (synthetic) colors
- Artificial (synthetic) flavors
- Antioxidant "BH" preservatives
- Salicylates

Stage Two
After observing a favorable response to Stage One, salicylates can be reintroduced one at a time and tested for tolerance. While some people find they need to remain on Stage One indefinitely, others are able to tolerate occasional salicylates, and some people can eat them freely. Many parents of ASD children see the biggest behavior improvements after removing salicylates. A Feingold mom quipped, "Feed him all the natural chocolate you want, but PLEASE don't feed him strawberries!"

Other items to consider eliminating:

- Corn Syrup
- MSG (Monosodium Glutamate)
- Nitrites or Nitrates
- Sulfiting agents
- Sulphur dioxide
- Sulfites
- Benzoates
- Phenols

Nambudripad's Allergy Elimination Techniques (NAET)

NAET is a method of treating allergies, ASD, ADD, and ADHD developed by the California physician, Dr. Devi Nambudripad MD (WI), D.C., L.Ac., Ph.D. (acu.). The diet is increasingly popular, and some of our patients have spoken positively of its benefits in combination with homeopathy. One of the main advantages of this therapy is that after NAET treatment, the child is able to be exposed to his allergens without reacting. Obviously, if treatment is successful, this is preferable to the enormous hassle of constantly avoiding and being on guard for potential allergen exposures.

NAET uses meridian acupressure points to clear allergies. After evaluating your child's allergens, a practitioner activates acupressure points with pressure or needles while the child holds the known allergen. Following treatment, patients wait for twenty minutes before being tested for muscle strength with the allergen in hand, a process known as applied kinesiology. If the allergen has been cleared, the theory goes, the child's arm should remain strong against the practitioner's pressure.

The parents are then instructed to ensure the child

avoids any contact with the treated allergen for twenty-five hours. Within seven days, the child should return to the practitioner's office to be re-tested for the treated allergen. If the allergen has been cleared, the practitioner then moves on to other allergens. Sometimes it takes more than one treatment to clear an allergen. In order to be considered successfully "cleared," the allergen should be at least 80-90% eliminated.

As with most therapies, there are pros and cons. We have heard positive feedback from a number of parents who have tried this method and found that many of their children's allergies had been eliminated. However, NAET addresses only one allergen per session, so it can be a time-consuming and costly process for children with multiple allergies.

Eliminating Mercury and Other Heavy Metals

As discussed earlier in Chapter 3, thimerosal, the mercury-based preservative used in vaccinations, has come under intense scrutiny. While this debate has yet to be resolved, the biochemical profile of autism frequently reveals heavy-metal toxicity, and the evidence for mercury as a causative factor is compelling.

Physiologically speaking, mercury has no place in the human body. It is toxic to all tissues and organs, and appears to have a specific affinity for nervous tissue. Unfortunately, environmental exposure to mercury continues to rise. In addition to dental amalgams (which are 50% mercury), fish such as swordfish and tuna usually contain significant mercury, so much so that pregnant women are now advised to limit their ingestion of tuna to no more than once a week. Until ten years ago, thimerosal was also used as a preservative agent in contact-lens solution.

Other potential heavy-metal exposures include

arsenic, lead, cadmium, and antimony. Arsenic is found in pressure-treated wood, some types of seafood, and sometimes in our drinking water. Lead is found in paint in older houses. Aluminum is found in cookware, drinking water, baking powder, and antiperspirants. Cadmium is released from cigarette smoke. Antimony is sometimes used as a flame retardant in carpets and children's pajamas. The best way to prevent heavy-metal toxicity is to avoid these exposures.

Several tests are available to determine levels of heavy metals. Hair analysis is the easiest and most cost-effective. However, mercury exposure will only be revealed in the hair if there has been a recent exposure. A DMSA challenge is another test commonly used to evaluate heavy-metal levels. With this method, a pre-challenge urine sample is obtained, then DMSA is administered. A post-challenge urine sample will then determine the presence of mercury.

Chelation therapy is the preferred method of removing mercury and other heavy metals from the body. Chelation agents such as DMPS, DMSA, EDTA, D-penicillamine and BAL bind the heavy metals, and usher them out of the body via the urine or stool. Chelation therapy is a specialized medical procedure, so it is essential to find someone qualified in this field if you choose to pursue this therapy.

Nutritional supplements that may also be helpful for detoxifying the body of mercury are cilantro, vitamin C, milk thistle, lipoic acid, selenium, N-acetylcysteine, and glycine. Some naturopathic doctors specialize in the detoxification of heavy metals and other environmental contaminants, using chelating substances and hydrotherapy, such as saunas followed by a cold plunge and alternating hot and cold applications.

Vitamin B6 and Magnesium

Vitamin B6 is essential to the operation of a majority of neurotransmitter pathways, including those for serotonin, dopamine, GABA, epinephrine and norepinephrine. Bernard Rimland, Ph.D., one of the foremost researchers on autism, pioneered the research and use of vitamin B6 and magnesium in children with autism. He conducted a meta-analysis of 18 studies involving vitamin B6 and magnesium.[62] All 18 studies demonstrated positive results with minimal side effects. Between 30 and 40% of the children showed significant improvement when B6 was given to them. He emphasizes, however, that the children were not "cured." Benefits included increased eye contact, more interest in surroundings, fewer self-stimming behaviors, fewer tantrums, and improved speech. More recently, Dr. Rimland conducted a study of over 200 autistic children, and half of the participants responded well to vitamin B6.

15

Bringing Balance To Your Family
Homeopathy for Parents and Siblings

Within a family, each individual plays a part in creating the family system. And like all living systems, families establish a balance called *homeostasis* whereby the other family members, as a whole, balance the qualities and characteristics of each individual family member.

If one person changes her role within a family, the rest of the system must change to re-establish balance. It's like a mobile hanging from the ceiling: if one portion of the mobile shifts position, the rest of the mobile must shift to regain equilibrium. The family system, as a whole, can move toward a state of health and adjustment. This is what can occur when a child with AS is successfully treated with homeopathy.

For example, if the mother of a family is over-functioning in terms of parenting responsibilities, it makes sense that her spouse might under-function within that role. If both over-functioned at the same time, the system would be out of balance. In another example, if a child with AS has special dietary needs, such as a GF/CF diet, this may demand extra energy on the part of the family cook. All of the effort and focus on that one child in the family will affect the other siblings and spouse, simply because of how time and attention are being allocated.

The rest of the family will respond to this, and attempt to find balance. As a result, while responding to one member of the family receiving increased attention, the spouse and siblings may feel angry, jealous, or unloved. This state can be unhealthy and disruptive.

Within family systems, we all develop established patterns and roles, especially when caring for a struggling family member. So, when a child with AS responds favorably to homeopathy or other interventions, it can move the whole system toward a state of overall health and well-being. Parents' roles will shift, responsibilities change, and the relationships within the family begin seeking a new balance.

The following cases are but two examples of how effectively treating parents and siblings can, both directly and indirectly, contribute to the health and well-being of a child with ASD.

Jemila: I Kept My Feelings All Inside

Jemila has been a patient of ours for five years, well before her son, Malik, came under our care for PDD. We have also treated her daughter for the past four years. Over the course of our therapeutic relationship, we have come to know Jemila very well. She will be the first to agree that homeopathic treatment has provided a much-needed support for her during an especially challenging period.

Jemila was 32 years old at the onset of treatment. Her major complaint at the time was a rash on her upper back. It was only after reading our book, *The Patient's Guide to Homeopathic Medicine,* that it became clear to Jemila there could be a connection between her skin problems and the emotional trauma she had experienced as a child. Migraines every couple of months were another concern.

> *When I was younger and living with my parents, I used to get frequent psychosomatic headaches with vomiting. I still clench my jaws and fists during my sleep. I have difficulty straightening out my hands when I first wake up. Warts also bother me. They disappeared for a long time and I have a small one on my pinky that's coming back.*
>
> *I would also like help with my mood swings. My anger becomes uncontrollable and I direct it all towards my husband. Now, with two young children, my patience is wearing thin. Lately I've been yelling more at my daughter. I just can't seem to get a handle on my emotions.*

Jemila was one of five siblings. Her father was busy with his chain of auto-parts stores and rarely at home. An extremely authoritarian man, he frequently yelled at his wife and kids. Jemila's mom, on the other hand, was a model of patience. Extremely sensitive by nature, Jemila would wilt when her father erupted in rage. Even though he never abused her physically, she was still afraid that he might when his temper flared. As a teen, she was diagnosed with TMJ. At times her jaw would lock, causing such pain that it was difficult for her to concentrate. Jemila still experienced jaw pain radiating down her neck, especially in cold weather.

> *My dad was highly controlling. Whenever I tried to express how I was feeling, my side of the argument, he'd shut me off. Even if I wanted to say something, I couldn't because it would make him even more furious. So I just held it in. I kept holding in*

*my feelings with him and with everyone else until I
met my husband. I think that's a lot of the cause of
my sickness. With my husband, I found myself subconsciously starting a fight, then shutting down. I
would lie there for hours, almost paralyzed. He
would try to get me to talk, but I would just freeze.
I know full well that it happened as a result of the
anger I couldn't get out with my father. I felt frozen.*

Her father made it clear that if she and her siblings
were not willing to do as he instructed, they should move
out of the house. Jemila ran away from home three or
four times, but always ended up, to her chagrin, going
back. She eventually extricated herself from the situation
by getting married, then moving to another state thousands of miles away from the family.

I See My Father in Myself
As much as Jemila intensely disliked her father's anger,
it was painful to recognize the very same tendency in
herself.

*I take out my aggression and negativity on my hus-
band. He tells me he can never please me. It's hard
for me to express my love to him. I think it's because
my parents never showed much affection to each
other or to me. I find myself perpetually nagging and
complaining and telling him the things he does
wrong. My patience with him is minimal. It's hard
with two kids. I simply don't have the time and
energy.*

In addition, she explained that her father's anger
"sensitized" her. If she found herself around friends who
treated their children abruptly, she experienced tightness

and stress in her body, just as she did as a child. When her husband yelled at their daughter about something she did wrong, Jemila would become disproportionately upset. It was as if she were reliving her childhood.

Once Jemila was at a friend's house and her little girl had accidentally pulled a flower out of the garden. The friend had a short fuse, in general, and the habit of screaming loudly at her child. She found herself anticipating the child's reaction, feeling it all through her body as if the woman were screaming at Jemila rather than her daughter. "I prepared myself for it. The mom ended up laughing about the whole thing." But Jemila couldn't stop her body from tensing up. With such a degree of sensitivity and tension, it was no wonder that she suffered from TMJ while living in the same house as her father.

Exceptional Features

 Jemila is a highly sensitive woman. What stood out the most in her initial interview was how damaged she had been by the atmosphere of anger in which she grew up. This reactivity became steadily more evident as we got to know her better. Jemila lived out her worst fear by internalizing her father's rage, expressing it only to her husband, with whom she felt safe and unafraid of being harmed, and, occasionally, to her children. Whenever she was around conflict or raised voices, the terror and indignation she experienced as a child was reactivated.

The medicine we prescribed initially, and which benefited Jemila for three years, was *Staphysagria* (stavesacre), a member of the *Ranunculaceae*, or buttercup, family. Those needing any of the plants in this family are highly sensitive to insult, humiliation, and unfair treatment. Refined and dignified, they do their best to keep their own anger under control. This exaggerated effort to suppress their rage can result in a variety of pathologies, most commonly urinary tract infections. In Jemila's case, her suppressed rage expressed itself in the form of boils. This was the first symptom that alerted that another dose of the *Staphysagria* was in order. These episodes occurred consistently after incidents in which she again suppressed her anger. Those needing this medicine often grow up in an environment where one parent is raging, dominant, and violent. For such a sensitive person, this is a terrifying situation.

Forgiving Her Father

Jemila waited five months before her first follow-up visit, and it was fortunate that she returned for support when she did. We soon learned that many of her physical complaints had improved since taking the initial dose of the medicine. Her tension headaches were better, and her jaw no longer locked. On a deeper level of healing, Jemila described how the *Staphysagria* had allowed her to forgive her parents. Able to finally realize how deeply the issues with her father had molded her life, she called upon her mother to help her with her healing. "For the first time, I want to confront my father. My mom told me, with great relief, that she had waited her entire life for the day when I told her what was wrong all along during my childhood. That day has finally come."

As often happens, however, a similar scenario emerged with a friend who Jemila considered powerful and authoritarian. This friend reminded Jemila of her father, and triggered some of the very same emotions.

I realize that I became a victim of her anger and frustration. It was exactly like when my father yelled at me as a kid. It affected me so profoundly I began to get psychosomatic attacks. I couldn't even function. I just lost it. Even taking care of the kids was too much. My relationship with my husband went out the door. I broke off the relationship with my friend. It was uncanny how everything about her is identical to my dad: her face, body motions, how she treats her kids. No wonder I felt so traumatized when I was little. And when I see how terribly sensitive my own daughter is! My mom says I was the spitting image of her.

I have so much more insight into my own patterns now. How I played the victim, held false beliefs, carried all this deep anger and resentment. I was able to talk it out with my mom. Watching myself get angry with the kids shows me how much it affects me.

Jemila received eight doses of the *Staphysagria* during her first three years of homeopathic care, sometimes following dental work which antidoted the medicine. Jemila became more keenly aware of things she had always wanted to express but never had, "shaping her entire perceptions of life."

When she was able, at last, to verbalize her feelings towards her father face to face, he genuinely apologized and explained the aspects of his own past that led him to behave as he did. Unburdened, Jemila's father was able to ask for her forgiveness. "I was very calm and took it nonchalantly. I told him I had already forgiven him."

For quite a while, Jemila continued to feel violated by her authoritarian friend, then those feelings diminished. Deeply spiritual prayer offered her great solace. Her relationship with her husband was up and down, but they continued to be committed to working on the marriage. Jemila's mood swings improved dramatically, recurring occasionally when she needed another dose of the

Staphysagria. The boils again erupted after highly emotionally charged events, though much less frequently.

Meeting the Demands of a Child with Pervasive Developmental Disorder

Less absorbed by her personal needs and those of a challenging marriage, Jemila devoted herself wholeheartedly to seeking out services for her son, Malik. As parents of ASD children are keenly aware, this can be a full-time endeavor. The family's limited finances made researching available resources even more compelling. Jemila's determination to leave no stone unturned in finding help for Malik placed quite a strain on the family, often leaving her daughter's and husband's needs unmet.

Jemila found the tremendous effort required for parenting a special-needs child to be exhausting—so exhausting that she began to "turn off" pain of any kind, physical or emotional. Jemila hit a low point. Everything in her life had become an ordeal. She was filled with a desire to escape, give up, to leave it all behind. Malik's needs, and those of her daughter, the marriage, everything—life all seemed too much to handle. Although Malik was progressing remarkably, the pressures of meeting his needs was taxing beyond belief. Doing it all, with no extended family to help was simply too much.

> *I no longer feel. My ability to feel is totally buried.*
> *I'm fighting for my son, my daughter, and me. The*
> *only way I can do that is to avoid listening to my*
> *own feelings. They slow me down. Just one more*
> *thing I have to handle. All my attention is focused on*
> *what I can do now to make things better for myself*
> *and my family. Considering what I'm dealing with,*
> *things have been going relatively well. Many other*
> *people would have lost it, and I have my moments of*

wondering if I will, too.

We asked Jemila to describe the feeling in her body that accompanied the recurrent boils: "It's like a needle getting poked into you—so sensitive. The pain can be so intense it's paralyzing. A sudden shock. Like when you slam your finger in a door."

She likened this feeling to how she felt during her father's raging outbursts:

> *That would paralyze me. Seeing how sensitive and tender my daughter is shows me exactly how I was. When he blew up, it would shake my world. Paralyze me. I would not be able to think or move. The same is happening now in dealing with my son. You never know when he'll have an outburst. Not knowing when this boil is going to erupt. It's a metal paralysis. I just can't think. The whole functioning of my brain is disorganized.*

These descriptions depicted her state of burnout and stagnancy, and the nearly superhuman effort needed to cope in her situation.

We changed Jemila' homeopathic medicine to *Helleborus* (black hellebore). Also a member of the buttercup family, it is used for individuals whose senses have been dulled to the extreme. This "shutting down" can be a coping mechanism; the person simply cannot handle the degree of sensitivity. A type of indifference or, as Jemila described her state, "numbness," results.

A Huge Difference
Jemila' six-week report was very positive:

> *I totally see a difference. My emotions are way more*

stable. I see now that there was a heavy, dark cloud looming over me that affected my thinking. The cloud has lifted. I'm more efficient in everything I do. Before, it took a huge effort to accomplish even daily tasks. It actually hurt to think. Even to sit down and plan a week's menu was painful. I was feeling so burnt out. Now I don't feel that way. My energy level is dramatically improved. My husband and I are doing much better together.

Four months later, Jemila shared,

I was able to get four months of respite care for Malik, but it's ending. We just finished a four-day assessment with him in another state. I have him on the simple-carbohydrate diet, so I need to cook everything ahead for the whole week. It is very stressful. A couple of days after we came back, I got a boil for the first time in six months. Other than that, my mental, emotional state has been stable. I feel strong and am taking things one step at a time. I'm doing so much better with handling life mentally and emotionally. When there are misunderstandings, it doesn't affect me in the way it did before. A lot of parents of special needs kids are on antidepressants. I think the only reason I'm not is because of the homeopathy.

We gave Jemila another dose of the *Helleborus*. Life, though immensely challenging, continues to be manageable for Jemila despite coping with her son's constant needs, the loss of her therapist, and her husband's entry into graduate school. Given the excessive demands with which she is dealing on an ongoing basis, she will need the support of homeopathy for some time.

Riley: I'm Not Gonna Do It!

You may remember Cody, the young man who was exquisitely fearful of and sensitive to being poked, cut, or stabbed. Cody's parents had also brought in his sister, Riley, for treatment. And it was a good thing they did, because straightening out Riley's behavior had a favorable impact on her brother's healing.

Riley exhibited a short fuse and manipulative tendencies. Her dad elaborated:

Her room is a tornado. She loves to dump out her drawers. We go through a major housecleaning once a week and she contributes to 99% of the mess. We tell her and her brother to pick it all up. Riley sits calmly on the bed, directing her brother to gather this and that, without lifting a finger. Then she laughs about it.

Our Riley has quite the temper. When she gets mad, she's furious. It takes no time at all for her to lash out and hit. Whoever it is that she's fighting with gets laid out.

Cody was playing outside with a sword and a shield. Riley grabbed a busted broom handle and went outside to play with him. I looked outside and her brother was crying as a result of a cut on his stomach where Riley had jabbed him. The following day, we received a call from the school principal, advising us that Riley had pummeled yet another child.

In the grand scheme of things, she's a sweetheart. She loves her brothers and will stand up for them, but she's downright lazy. All she wants to do is create messes, huge messes, but she wants nothing to do with cleaning them up afterwards. You wouldn't believe what Riley does with our dresser. The

little stinker has gutted the entire room, swept every-
thing on top of the dresser onto the floor, then stood
there admiring her work. Then she actually denies
having done it despite all the telltale signs that she's
guilty. Riley comes up with the most outlandish,
unbelievable excuses like, 'One of the upstairs kids
did it.' One night I asked her to go get the silverware
for the dinner table. She yelled back at me, 'I'm not
gonna do it. I do everything!' She went without din-
ner that night.

If Riley's mood turned sour, she was quick to
kick the dog or crouch on all fours under the table
swinging to hit him. Or she would smack him on the
rear and scream 'Stupid dog!' "It's like she's blind
with rage," her father said, "We keep telling her to
leave the dog alone. Riley does the same thing with
her brother. She'll keep coming at him until she
makes physical contact with him, even if he attempts
to dodge her.

Her Way or the Highway

Riley's run-ins with authority occurred not only at home,
but at school as well. When this little girl's mind was
made up, there was no changing it. Nobody could make
her do anything; it was "her way or the highway." This
little girl earned the nickname "Queen of the Sandbox."
The father explained that Riley was so set in her ways
that, no matter what the consequence, she wouldn't
budge. "I tell her to clean up her room and Riley answers,
'Why?' I tell her, 'Because I'm you're daddy.' And she
replies, 'You're not my daddy!' I tell her to get in the car
and she screams, 'It's not my car!'"

If she didn't feel like doing an assignment, Riley
scribbled over it. The year before, Riley left class in a huff
and walked out to the playground. A couple of other

times, she simply ducked out of school and walked home for no apparent reason except that she felt like it. Riley's parents had figured out that it didn't matter how big or authoritative they were. The only way to get Riley to cooperate was to recognize that *she* was the boss.

Riley had suffered quite a few bouts of vaginal yeast from age five on, sometimes to the point where walking became painful. Antifungal cream had helped somewhat. She had shown a tendency to masturbate from a very early age, and bedwetting was still a periodic issue.

The Big Chill

Now it was our turn to experience Riley's steadfast determination. Usually, at this point in an initial case taking, we speak directly with the child, usually for thirty to sixty minutes. We prefer to do this without the parent(s) present whenever possible, extending the same privacy to kids that we do to adults. Riley's dad brought her into the interviewing room. She took one defiant look at us, sat down in the chair directly facing us, and there she sat, silent for the next thirty minutes. We tried every trick we knew to get her to interact with us—even offering her some delectable Swiss chocolate, which her father had already told us she adored. She ignored the chocolate entirely and spoke not a single word. Score another point for Riley.

Exceptional Features

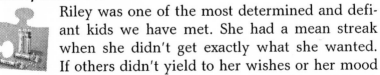
Riley was one of the most determined and defiant kids we have met. She had a mean streak when she didn't get exactly what she wanted. If others didn't yield to her wishes or her mood turned angry, Riley thought nothing of punching siblings, animals, classmates, or whoever made her mad. We have met a few kids who decided not to speak during the

interview. But none had Riley's arrogance and satisfaction.

This chronic attitude, combined with the recurring vaginal infections and tendency to masturbate led us to first prescribe *Medorrhinum* (a nosode), which helped her only temporarily.

At the first follow-up telephone consultation, we changed to *Platina* (platinum) with a very positive outcome. *Platina* is an excellent medicine for girls with superior attitudes who suffer from vaginal complaints. These girls are also typically sexually precocious. It fit the bill for Riley, who was six years old going on sixteen.

Baby PMS

Riley's parents did not schedule a second phone consultation for five months. Riley's tantrums had subsided for two months after taking the *Platina*, but then returned. The rocking on the floor to masturbate, quite frequent previously, had decreased considerably. Riley was still demanding, though to a lesser degree. Still prone to tantrums and mood swings, her mom referred to Riley's sudden mood fluctuations as "baby PMS."

> *We never know. It's really scary. She'll have some incident that incenses her, then she won't speak. If Riley is at school, she absolutely will not go to the lunchroom or do anything she's told. I'm her mother and I live with her, and I still can't figure her out. If I try to talk to her, it makes it worse. I go through a gamut of questioning and she won't even answer. Riley's moods are so unpredictable.*

Her mom also emphasized how overly sensitive Riley was to being examined vaginally by her pediatrician, "screaming bloody murder" even during a well-child exam. Even with a woman doctor, she could not tolerate the least touch, due to the sensitivity of the inflamed area.

Much More Cooperative

At this point, looking for a more significant change in Riley's moods and mistreatment of her brother, we gave her a higher dose of *Platina*. Two months later, the report was very positive. Her aggression towards her brother had diminished markedly, and Riley was much more cooperative—a quantum leap from how she had been before. She and her brother had enjoyed an unusually harmonious summer together. The family even traveled together by car without any memorable incidents, quite a feat considering how things had been.

Riley needed a repetition of the *Platina* after a regression in crankiness, self-stimulatory rocking, and vaginal irritation. One other dose of the medicine was given more recently, after Riley slathered her lips in Carmex, a camphor and menthol-containing lip balm known to interrupt the action of homeopathic medicines in some cases. As long as the *Platina* is acting, this young lady is much easier on her brother, her parents, and anyone who crosses her path. Homeopathic treatment for Riley has lightened the family's load a great deal and, thankfully, taken pressure off Cody. Riley has even agreed to talk to us during her next appointment. Now that's progress!

16

Practical Tips for Living With and Learning From Your Child with ASD

❧ *Love, First and Foremost*
Absolutely the most important thing you can do to help your child with ASD is to open your heart and tell your child you love him. Again and again. No matter whether he talks to you, or even looks you in the eyes. Even when he throws tantrums, rages, or breaks your most precious possessions. Whether his grades are As or Fs. Even if he spaces out on the soccer field, kicks the ball into the other team's goal, and appears to make a total fool out of himself, over and over. Regardless of whether he tells you the same facts about trains or cube roots for the 200th time that day. The bottom line is that what matters the most is that you love him.

❧ *Take One Moment at a Time*
You may have heard the expression "chunk down." It means taking life in small, manageable, bite-size pieces. As a parent of a child with ASD, you probably feel over the top most of the time, with more responsibilities than any two people could successfully fulfill, yet never feeling like you are doing enough, giving enough, or finishing enough.

Your child has so many needs and time always seems short. Your conscientiousness in taking care of your family is admirable, but are you so busy preparing for tomorrow that you completely miss the magic of right now? Stop for just one minute, look around, take a deep breath, and simply be *right here, right now*. You might even want to use a few words to remind yourself to be in the moment, such as, "Breathe in, breathe out" or "I'm okay here and now."

❧ Tomorrow is Another Day

Maybe you're an organized, efficient list maker who cannot possibly accomplish half of what you expect of yourself each day. Or maybe you can't even get as far as making the list! Be realistic about what you *can* do each day, given all that's on your plate. Be easy on yourself. Tackle what must be done today—tasks that will have negative consequences if postponed until tomorrow. These tasks might be things like getting your kids up, cleaned, fed, dressed, and to school on time (unless you homeschool), or paying the overdue phone or gas bill.

But lots of other tasks will fall into the "wouldn't it be nice if?" category. You have every intention of getting them done, but the sky will not fall in if they wait another day or week. At the end of each day, give yourself credit for what you *did* do, go to sleep with a clear mind, then get up fresh to meet the next day.

❧ You and Your Child Are Both Doing the Best You Can

It's easy to criticize; it's much more challenging to give each other the benefit of the doubt. The minute we honestly recognize and acknowledge that, no matter how we or our kids screw up, we really are trying our best, everything lightens up a bit.

Children with ASD have a different take on the world, and we have much to learn from them. We cannot, nor should we, expect these kids to think, act, function, reason, or behave like NTs. Nor should they. The more you practice repositioning yourself, and making a sincere attempt to understand the world from your child's eyes, the more that world will make sense to you, or at least will seem less foreign. If your child is hypersensitive to noise, think about how easy it would be for you to concentrate on homework or conversation with blaring music going all the time. If your child has tactile sensitivities, remind yourself of just how annoying a pebble in your shoe can be, and multiply that by ten. If constant discussion of the same subject is bugging you, try to remember a time when *you* felt such wonder and delight in a topic, and relive that wonder through your child's "grand passion."

In some ways, your child's view of the world might even make more sense than the way the rest of society is adapting and living. We highly recommend the delightful and instructive novel, *The Curious Incident of the Dog in the Night-Time*, by Mark Haddon, which provides one of the best opportunities we know of to climb inside the mind of an adolescent with ASD.

❦ *Allow Your Child to Be Himself*
There is no other child in the world as lovable as *your* child, inscrutable, and impossible as he might sometimes be. You may not be happy with everything he does. You may even have sinking moments, wondering why you ever became a parent in the first place.

Without the quirks and oddities that make each of us who we are, life would be no more than varying shades of gray. Consider the diversity that comes from a rainbow of personalities, habits, and worldviews.

Be grateful for the many ways in which your child contributes so beautifully to this diversity. We interviewed a child the other day who stated the matter quite succinctly: "Why would I want to be like everyone else? That would be totally boring. I love being different."

❧ Be Proactive About Your Child's Diagnosis and Treatment

Being parents of children with ASD, you hardly need encouragement to be proactive. We have never seen a more involved, motivated, and determined group of parents. As you well know, you cannot necessarily depend on your child's teacher, physicians, or other caregivers to advocate for your child. A passive approach to meeting these children's needs rarely bears fruit. Whether it means seeking out funding for respite care or special interventions, researching and locating therapeutic resources, or finding the best blend of conventional and alternative medicine, your efforts largely determine how far and how quickly your child progresses.

It can take several years to reach a diagnosis. In some cases, the child is a young adult before all the pieces fall together. The earlier you press for a comprehensive assessment, the sooner you can put together an intervention strategy. The more involved you are in seeking out the best care for your child, including homeopathy, the better your child's outcome is likely to be.

With the wealth of ASD resources now available through books, the Internet, support groups, and elsewhere, you can quickly become an ASD "expert." The more you know about the diagnosis, possible causes, treatment options, and resources available, the more powerful an advocate you can be for your child. Understanding terms such as theory of mind, NT, and Aspie, can be enlightening. The more knowledgeable you are about ASD, the more conversant you can be with doctors, teachers, and other care providers, and the more you can make educated choices about medication, education, and therapeutic interventions. If and when specific causes of ASD are identified and verified, you will be among the first to know and, can respond accordingly. By keeping up with the latest advances and treatment approaches, you can also spread the word to other parents who can, in turn, do the same.

❦ *Be Consistent with Discipline*

Confer and strategize with your partner, or others involved in parenting your child, to develop a style of discipline that works for your child and for you. Kids need clear and consistent limits, plain and simple. Mixed messages are confusing. If your child's behavior is inappropriate, let him know *at the time* what is expected of him. Set fair consequences, and be willing to enforce them.

Modeling positive behaviors for your child with ASD can only improve his chances of making friends and gaining attention appropriately. Consistency in setting ground rules is even more essential in large, blended families, or divorced families, where the chaos factor can be especially hard for a child with ASD to bear.

If you find yourself losing it, use whatever techniques are necessary to pull yourself back together. Give yourself a friendly reminder that you've been through this before, and you'll make it through again. In a quiet moment alone (we know they're rare!), examine your patterns. Take a close look at situations that push you to your limit. If you can better understand what's going on during a "cooler" time, you'll be more likely to act the way you'd like in the heat of the moment. And remember to go easy on yourself!

❦ *The Son Rise Approach*

On a different note, sometimes discipline isn't a response that will elicit the most optimal outcome, particularly with self-stimming and perseverative behaviors. Another option is taught by the Son Rise program developed by Barry Neil Kaufman (see Appendix). Son Rise emphasizes *joining* in your child's repetitive and ritualistic behaviors in a nonjudgmental and loving manner. *Joining*, as opposed to suppressing or disciplining, is actually quite close to the homeopathic principle of *like cures like*.

❦ *Nurture Family Dynamics*

Living with a special-needs child can strain an already delicate family system. Adding hours of therapy, special meal preparation, and medical care to an already full family schedule makes for frayed nerves all around. It is inevitable that tension and resentments will arise, so it's important to keep the lines of communication flowing rather than stifling your emotions. Regular family meetings are one way to give each family member an opportunity to express his or her feelings openly. Family meetings can create a nurturing and safe environment in which all family members can really listen to each other and be heard. Be sure to include your child with ASD, so that he feels like an integral member of the family. In addition to creating special occasions for everyone in the family to enjoy each other together, set aside individual time to do something fun with your spouse and the other children.

❦ *Be Your Child's Strongest Supporter*

Do not for a moment give up on your child. We have seen miracles with ASD children. It is your belief in your child that will convince her she can do anything, whether or not she can communicate that belief to you. Kevin, the teenager whose story is told earlier in this book, expressed to his mother how glad he was that she kept searching out avenues of healing for him. Even if you are surrounded by disapproval or judgment, hold on to your conviction that your child will find the programs, health-care providers, and support that he needs. Be relentless in cheering him on, even when you are the only one there for him. Your standing by him, no matter what, will reap rich rewards. Years from now, you'll be able to look back and see you left no stone unturned to help your child become all that he could.

❦ Ally With Other Parents and Families

The resources available for you to connect with, learn from, and get support from other ASD parents are remarkable. The OASIS website is a shining example of this! But there are also support groups and networks springing up nationwide. Take advantage of the wisdom of others who have gone through the process before you. Despite how it may feel day to day, you are *not* alone. There are many other parents who have one or more children with ASD and other special needs who have walked a very similar path to yours. Let them hold your hand or give you a lift up the road when you need it, and you can do the same for others.

PART FIVE

Exploring Homeopathic Treatment More Fully

17

The Most Common Questions Asked by Parents of Children with ASD

❧ *How Do I Know if Homeopathy Can Help My Child?*

If your child has AS, or is on the milder end of the autism spectrum, it is quite likely that homeopathy can help. If your child has autistic disorder or is non-verbal, success depends on several factors: the relevant experience of the homeopath, the severity of disability of your child, and your level of motivation. Sometimes it is helpful to speak with the practitioner before scheduling to get an idea how familiar he is with ASD. While each patient is considered a unique individual to the homeopath, it is undeniable that experience counts.

Some children, regardless of their diagnoses, are virtually "textbook" as far as matching a homeopathic symptom picture. Other youngsters are more challenging and may require trials with a number of medicines before the correct one is found. A homeopath can give you a better idea of her level of confidence about your child's treatment prognosis at the conclusion of the initial case taking. The definitive answer as to whether homeopathy will be an effective treatment for *your* youngster can only be given after the child has been in treatment for six months to a year.

❦ *How Much Can Homeopathy Help My Child?*
This again depends on a number of factors, including how severely disabled your child is, and whether the homeopath can find a medicine that matches her symptoms very well. If your child is on the milder end of the spectrum, such as AS, our experience is that homeopathy can help significantly, even to the point of academic mainstreaming, dramatic behavioral changes, and impressive social interactions. We have had some AS parents use the word "normal" to describe their children after homeopathic care.

Rest assured that homeopathy will not take away the positive features of your child that make her who she is, but will rather bring into balance anything that interferes with her health, happiness, and functioning in life. Because the autism spectrum is so wide, we hesitate to give any numbers regarding percentage of improvement. However, in the case of children with ADHD, we generally expect a 70% or greater improvement if the child continues treatment for at least a year. Additionally, we can certainly say that, if your child benefits from homeopathy, everyone will notice—you, grandparents, teachers, friends, caregivers. The difference is marked and clearly recognizable.

❦ *What About "Lower-Functioning" Children with ASD?*
Homeopathy has the potential to treat more severely autistic children. The biggest problem can be the inability of the child to communicate verbally. However, this is not always an insurmountable obstacle since we do not actually speak with some of our other pediatric patients either, because they are too young, too shy, or for some

other reason. If there is no speech, we rely more on our own and the parents' observations of the child's movements, facial expressions, and gestures. There are parents who know their children so well and are such articulate reporters that they give us all the information we need in order to prescribe effectively. Some parents are less able to provide the objective information that is useful to a homeopath in the initial interview. Over the course of homeopathic interviews, though, they learn which information we are likely to find most useful. Regardless of exactly where a child is on the spectrum, when the right medicine is found, the transformation can be remarkable.

❦ Will Phone Consultations Work for My Child?

Many homeopaths see patients only in person. We have developed a phone practice, in addition to the patients we see in person, because there are relatively few homeopaths throughout the United States, especially those specializing in treating children with mental, emotional, developmental, and behavioral problems. We have found that our twenty-plus years of experience generally make up for what may be lost by not seeing the child in person, although we encourage parents to bring their children to see us for at least the first appointment if possible. Even if the first interview is conducted by phone, it is possible to visit us in person later in the treatment process.

Just as a blind person learns to cultivate other senses, so we find that we listen in other ways and that our results are generally as good with phone patients as with our local patients. In fact, when we present our best teaching cases at seminars or conferences, we notice that they often turn out to be our long-distance patients.

We do ask all patients, local or long-distance, to send us a photograph. We welcome video clips, and we are looking into the use of video-conferencing over the Internet.

❧ *Can Homeopathy Help Adults with ASD?*

Although the thrust of this book is ASD children, the information and guidelines apply equally to adults. No one is too old to begin homeopathic treatment. Homeopathy treats the whole person, adult or child, and can address the ASD adult's physical, mental, and emotional complaints, as well as problems related to work, relationships, communication, and sensitivities.

❧ *Does Homeopathic Medicine Have Side Effects?*

Homeopathic medicines are prepared by a process of serial dilution that leaves only an imprint of the original substance remaining in the medicine. This explains why even poisons, such as arsenic and strychnine, can be made into homeopathic preparations with absolutely no risk of toxicity. Homeopathic medicines do not produce side effects like those of prescription, or even over-the-counter, medications. They are natural and nontoxic, and, because of the serial dilutions, are actually far safer even than herbs, much less pharmaceutical drugs.

As we mentioned earlier, sometimes people will have an aggravation period when symptoms temporarily worsen before getting much better. A less frequent phenomenon is a return of old symptoms during the course of treatment, which lasts three or four days, before disappearing for good. An aggravation and return of old symptoms typically occur only after the correct medicine is given.

One other reaction is a proving, in which a patient who takes the same homeopathic medicine over and over begins to develop new symptoms he did not have before. We rarely see this in our practice, but the symptoms abate as soon as the medicine is discontinued.

❦ My Child is Highly Sensitive or Vaccine-Damaged. Is Homeopathy Safe for Such a Child?

Only you can decide what you feel comfortable with for your child. Homeopathy is probably the safest of all types of medication, yet a highly sensitive child can react even to our medicine. If you let us know, before we prescribe the indicated homeopathic medicine, that your child is extremely reactive or sensitive we can select the proper potency of the medicine to use. To diminish even those relatively few reactions that a child can experience, we can prescribe a lower potency medicine, use an LM (fifty-thousand dilutions) preparation, or use a double-glass method of dilution.

❦ Can Homeopathy be Combined with Psychiatric or Other Medications?

Yes. Some of our patients are taking conventional medications, such as psychotropic drugs, when they begin homeopathic treatment. Sometimes as improvement occurs it is possible, under the guidance of the prescribing physician, to decrease the dosage of or discontinue these medicines. There are some prescription drugs that need to be taken for life, though this is less true with children.

Homeopathic medicines cannot interfere with the action of conventional pharmaceuticals. Because some prescription medications, particularly steroids and long-term antibiotics, can suppress the immune systems or suppress or mask symptoms, it is important that your homeopath know about any medications prescribed for your child.

❦ How Does a Homeopath Decide What to Give My Child?

A classical homeopath bases the decision of which medicine to give your child on a lengthy interview with parent(s) and child. You will be asked to fill out a medical history form and provide information from teachers, other providers, and caregivers. Additionally, psychological and educational assessments can be helpful. You may want to inquire first just what information to send, however, since we have at times received far more extensive notes than we need. Practitioners choosing homeopathic medicines based on electronic machines, muscles testing, pendulums, radionics, or methods other than an in-depth interview are not using the classical homeopathy that we are describing and recommending in this book.

❦ How Long Does it Take to Notice the Positive Effects of a Homeopathic Medicine?

Depending on whether your child receives a single dose or daily dose of medicine, you should notice a difference within one to four weeks. There may be an initial, brief worsening of symptoms, called an aggravation. After a few days, the symptoms should steadily improve. After your child has become stabilized on the medicine, the positive changes should be lasting. Of course, there will always be some ups and downs due to the stresses and adjustments demanded by everyday life. This new and improved state of being should last until, either because of interference or the passage of time, the homeopathic medicine needs to be repeated.

❦ How Frequent are Appointments?

Frequency of appointments varies somewhat among practitioners, but, typically, appointments are six to eight weeks apart initially, then every three to four months as the child gets better. It is necessary to allow enough time to elapse after a dose of the medicine is given to thoroughly assess its effect. The same frequency is true of phone consultations.

❦ How Long Will My Child Need Homeopathic Treatment?

With ASD, plan on continuing treatment for a minimum of one to two years. If you are happy with the results, you will probably want to continue with homeopathic care long-term as well as having the other members of your family treated.

❦ How Do I Know if Other Family Members Should be Treated as Well?

Rare is the individual, child or adult, who cannot benefit from homeopathic treatment to some degree, especially given the stresses and strains of living with and caring for a special-needs child. Although you may rise swiftly to the occasion, apparently coping to beat the band, you may be quietly fraying around the edges. The same may be true of your spouse or co-parent, and for siblings who may experience, openly or silently, their share of disappointment, resentment, and jealousy. It is wonderful to see how much more smoothly families can function when everyone is receiving homeopathic treatment. Read Chapter 16 to learn more about the benefits of treating the whole family with homeopathy.

❦ How Are Acute Illnesses Managed During Homeopathic Treatment?

Depending on the severity of the illness and the proximity and availability of your homeopath, there are several choices of courses to follow. If possible, and the situation is not urgent, call you homeopath first for advice. Homeopathy can be rapidly and amazingly effective for many acute illnesses, as well as first-aid situations. If your homeopath is not available, the condition is urgent, or your homeopath instructs you to do so, consult a local physician for a diagnosis and, possibly, treatment.

Many of our patients have on hand our book, *Homeopathic Self-Care: The Quick and Easy Guide for the Whole Family* and the companion home medicine kit. The book is filled with homeopathic and naturopathic advice for self-care of 70 acute and first-aid conditions. If you do seek out conventional treatment for an acute illness, be sure to notify your homeopath as soon as possible afterwards so she can record the information in your child's chart, make appropriate recommendations, and, if appropriate, give your child an acute or constitutional medicine.

❦ *What is the Cost of Homeopathic Treatment?*

Cost of homeopathic care is highly variable depending on the following factors: training, degree, and licensure of the practitioner; board certification; experience; length of office visits; and location. If you are comparing the cost of homeopathic versus conventional treatment, it is important to know the length of each visit, since a first appointment for a child in our practice lasts two hours. Practitioners with similar credentials and experience are likely to charge much more than a homeopath with no formal medical training. Fees vary enormously—the highest we know of being $2,000 for a first visit and the lowest, $200. In general, $1,500 should easily cover the first year of treatment, excluding any additional nutritional supplements. Homeopathic medicines themselves cost so little as to be virtually free, especially in comparison with psychotropic medications.

❦ *How Can I Find a Qualified Homeopathic Doctor or Practitioner?*

Make sure the prospective homeopath is well trained and experienced in classical homeopathy, and is at least certified, if not board certified, in homeopathic medicine. We recommend a homeopath whose practice is at least 75%

homeopathy and who participates actively in continuing homeopathic education. When choosing a naturopathic doctor, make sure the individual graduated from a reputable four-year naturopathic medical college and is a board certified diplomate. It is wise, in the case of children on the autism spectrum, to choose a practitioner well versed in treating children with psychiatric problems. The more experience that person has had in treating children with ASD, the better, although there are as yet very few of us who have seen any significant number of kids in this population. For more information, see Chapter 6 and the Homeopathic Resources section of the Appendix.

❦ What is the Difference Between Receiving Professional Homeopathic Care and Buying the Medicines at a Pharmacy or Health Food Store?

Single or combination homeopathic medicines are becoming increasingly available even in neighborhood pharmacies. These medicines are commonly in 30C potencies or lower, not as strong as your homeopath would typically use. Such products may be helpful in self-treatment for acute illnesses, but we discourage self-treatment for chronic conditions such as ASD, depression, irritable bowel syndrome, eczema, or allergies. You would not go to a pharmacy to buy bandages so that you could perform minor surgery on your child. In the same way, treatment of chronic conditions should be left to professionals.

❦ Can I Combine Other Therapies with Homeopathy?

Yes, many other therapies are quite compatible with homeopathy. Discuss with your homeopath any adjunctive therapies you are pursuing or considering. He may ask that, once a new homeopathic medicine is prescribed, you wait a couple of months before introducing a new intervention in order to adequately evaluate the effect of the homeopathy. Adding too many therapies at the same time can make it confusing to know to what extent each of them is working. Most therapeutic modalities that are already being used before beginning homeopathy are likely to be fine to continue, depending on the advice of the individual homeopath.

❧ Can Homeopathy be Combined with a GF/CF, SCD™, Feingold, or a Hypoallergenic Diet?

Yes. Many of the ASD children we treat are already on one of these diets just as a number of our ADHD patients have benefited from the Feingold Diet. If you are not aware of your child's nutritional needs, feel free to discuss this with us so that we can make recommendations. Simply increasing the amount and frequency of protein in a child's diet can make a big difference in behavior.

❧ Can Nutritional Supplements Complement Homeopathy?

Being naturopathic as well as homeopathic doctors, we are strong believers in a healthy diet and high-quality nutritional supplementation. Supplements can be extremely effective supportively to keep ASD children healthy. We are continually looking for the best new natural products on the market.

We have an extensive naturopathic pharmacy that is used secondarily to homeopathy. One difference with a homeopath, however, is that you will not be given a shopping bag full of supplements, but rather a few, since the correct homeopathic medicine should address *all* of a child's problems.

❧ *Do Insurance Providers Cover Homeopathic Care?*

The best bet is to check with your insurance provider. The third-party payer scenario has changed dramatically and promises to continue to do so, making it difficult to generalize about coverage of homeopathy. Homeopathic medicine is not a licensed profession, so the licensure depends on the medical degree of the practitioners, whether ND, MD, DO, etc. In certain states, naturopathic physicians, acupuncturists, and even certified, unlicensed homeopaths are covered by insurance. Even if you are not reimbursed, the care may be included in your out-of-pocket deductible. Since homeopathic visits, particularly the initial case taking, are much longer than most insurance providers allot, even if your practitioner is covered, the full cost of the first visit may not be. The same is true for telephone consultations.

Appendix
Resources for ASD, Homeopathy, Diets, and Vaccination Information

Autism Spectrum Disorder (ASD)

Attwood, Tony. *Asperger's Syndrome.* London: Jessica Kingsley Publishers, 1998.

Frith, Uta (Editor). *Autism and Asperger's Syndrome.* Cambridge: Cambridge University Press, 1991.

Grandin, Temple. *Thinking in Pictures.* New York: Doubleday, 1995.

Grandin, Temple and Scarimo, Margaret. *Emergence: Labeled Autistic.* New York, Warner Books, 1996.

Gray, Carol. *Comic Strip Conversations.* Arlington, TX: Future Horizons, 1994.

Haddon, Mark. *The Curious Incident of the Dog in the Night-Time,* New York, NY: Vintage, 2004.

Willey, Liane Holliday. *Pretending to be Normal: Living with Asperger's Syndrome.* London: Jessica Kingsley Publishers, 1999.

Bashe, Patricia Romanowski and Kirby, Barbara L. *The OASIS Guide to Asperger Syndrome.* New York, NY: Crown Publishing, 2001.

Seroussi, Karyn. *Unraveling the Mystery of Autism & PDD: A Mother's Story of Research and Recovery.* New York, NY: Simon and Schuster, 2000.

Myles, Brenda Smith. *Asperger Syndrome and Difficult Moments.* Shawnee Mission, KS: Autism Asperger Publishing Company, 2001.

www.aspergersyndrome.org
The OASIS website is an outstanding and utterly invaluable resource.
www.aspergersyndrome.com
Clinical psychologist Sally Bloch-Rosen's website. Oriented for professionals, educators, and parents alike.

www.autism.org
The Center for the Study of Autism website.

www.isn.net/~jypsy/
Oops! Wrong Planet Website. A website created by a family for families affected by ASD.

www.latitudes.org
Bi-monthly newsletter of the Alternative Therapy Network devoted to alternative therapies for ADD, TS and autism.

www.thegraycenter.org
The website of Carol Gray, director of the Gray Center for Social Learning and Understanding.   ·

www.son-rise.org
The Autism Treatment Center of America's Son Rise program website.

Homeopathy

Bellavite, Paolo and Signorini, Andrea. *The Emerging Science of Homeopathy: Complexity, Biodynamics, and Nanopharmacology.* Berkeley, CA: North Atlantic Books, 2002.
Castro, Miranda. *The Complete Homeopathy Handbook: A Guide to Everyday Healthcare.* New York, NY: St. Martin's Press, 1991.
Castro, Miranda. *Homeopathy for Pregnancy, Birth and Your Baby's First Year,* New York, NY: St. Martin's Press, 1997.

Cummings, Stephen, and Ullman, Dana. *Everybody's Guide to Homeopathic Medicines: Safe and Effective Medicines for You and Your Family* (3rd ed.). Los Angeles, CA: J.P. Tarcher, 1980.

Gray, Bill. *Homeopathy: Science or Myth?* Berkeley, CA: North Atlantic Books, 2002.

Hahnemann, Samuel. *Organon of the Medical Art* (Edited by Wenda Brewster O'Reilly). Redmond, WA: Birdcage Books, 1996.

Jonas, Wayne and Jacobs, Jennifer. *Healing with Homeopathy.* New York, NY: Warner Books, 1996.

Lansky, Amy. *Impossible Cure: The Promise of Homeopathy.* Portola, CA: R.L. Ranch Press, 2003.

Reichenberg-Ullman, Judyth and Ullman, Robert. *The Patient's Guide to Homeopathic Medicine.* Edmonds, WA: Picnic Point Press, 1995.

Reichenberg-Ullman, Judyth and Ullman, Robert. *Homeopathic Self Care: The Quick and Easy Guide for the Whole Family,* Prima Publishing, 1997.

Reichenberg-Ullman, Judyth and Ullman, Robert. *Prozac Free.* Berkeley, CA: North Atlantic Books, 2001.

Reichenberg-Ullman, Judyth and Ullman, Robert. *Rage-Free Kids.* Edmonds, WA: Picnic Point Press, 2003.

Reichenberg-Ullman, Judyth and Ullman, Robert. *Ritalin-Free Kids* (2nd ed). Rocklin, CA: Prima Publishing, 2000.

Ullman, Dana. *The Consumer's Guide to Homeopathic Medicine.* New York, NY: Tarcher/Putnam, 1995.

www.drugfreeasperger.com
Drs. Reichenberg-Ullman, Ullman, and Luepker's site for the homeopathic treatment of Asperger Syndrome. This site also provides access to information about all of our other books, kits, speaking schedule, and services.

www.homeopathicdirectory.com
A certifying organization for classical homeopaths in Canada and the United States.

www.healthy.net/HANP
The Homeopathic Academy of Naturopathic Physicians
(HANP)—directory of naturopathic physicians board certified
in homeopathy.

www.homeopathic.com
Homeopathic Educational Services—homeopathic books,
tapes, and other educational resources.

www.homeopathic.org
The National Center for Homeopathy (NCH) website—the
primary homeopathic organization in the United States.

www.homeopathy.org
The North American Society of Homeopaths (NASH)
represents all certified homeopaths in North America.

www.minimum.com
Minimum Price Books—a source for homeopathic books,
tapes, and products.

ASD and Diet

Gottschall, Elaine Gloria. *Breaking the Vicious Cycle: Intestinal
    Health Through Diet*. Ontario, Canada: Kirkton Press, 1994.
Lewis, Lisa. *Special Diets for Special Kids*. Arlington, TX:
    Future Horizons, 1998.

www.autismndi.com
A site for information regarding GF/CF diets.

www.breakingtheviciouscycle.info
Elaine Gloria Gottschall's website on dietary intervention.

www.feingold.org
The Feingold Program website.

Vaccination Information

Cave, Stephanie., Mitchell, Deborah. *What Your Doctor May Not Tell You About Children's Vaccinations.* New York, NY: Warner Books, 2001.

Neustaedter, Randall. *The Vaccine Guide: Making An Informed Choice.* Berkeley, CA: North Atlantic Books, 1995.

Glossary

acute illness—a condition that is self-limiting and short-lived, generally lasting only a few days to a couple of months

aggravation—a temporary worsening of already existing symptoms after taking a homeopathic medicine

antidote—a substance or influence that interferes with homeopathic treatment

attention deficit disorder (ADD)—synonymous with ADHD

attention-deficit/hyperactivity disorder (ADHD)—a diagnosis based on a constellation of symptoms that includes hyperactivity, attention problems, and/or impulsivity

AS—see Asperger syndrome

aspie—a term preferred by some with AS to denote Asperger syndrome

Asperger syndrome (AS)—a neurological disorder affecting social interaction and communication which is accompanied by a restricted, stereotyped and repetitive pattern of behaviors, interests, and activities

ASD—see autism spectrum disorder

autism spectrum disorder (ASD)—includes the wider spectrum of autistic disorders, from low to high-functioning

case taking—the process of the in-depth homeopathic interview

casein—the primary protein in cow's milk

central auditory processing disorder (CAPD)—inability of individuals with normal hearing and intelligence to differentiate, recognize, or understand sounds

classical homeopathy—a method of homeopathic prescribing in which only one medicine is given at a time, based on the totality of the patient's symptoms

constitutional treatment—homeopathic treatment based on the whole person, involving an extensive interview and careful follow-up

conventional medicine—mainstream Western medicine that follows orthodox views of diagnosis and treatment

developmental disability (DD)—mental or physical delays in development and maturity due to genetic or congenital abnormalities; previously called mental retardation

DSM-IV—the diagnostic and statistical manual, published by the American Psychological Association, which classifies mental and emotional disorders into diagnostic categories

echolalia—repetition or parroting of words or phrases, usually with little or no comprehension

FDA—United States Food and Drug Administration

Feingold Diet—a dietary approach for treating ASD that involves the elimination of food colorings, additives, preservatives, flavorings, and salicylates

gluten—a protein in grains such as wheat, oats, rye, and barley

high potency homeopathic medicines—medicines of a 200C potency or higher

homeopathic medicine—a medicine that acts according to the principles of homeopathy

homeopathy—the use of a substance that causes a particular set of symptoms in a healthy person to relieve similar symptoms in a person who is ill

hyperlexia—heightened, and often precocious, literacy skills without comprehension

Law of Similars—the medical concept, which dates back to Hippocrates, that like cures like

learning disability (LD)—an umbrella term referring to group of disorders characterized by significant difficulties in the acquisition and use of listening, spelling, reading, writing, reasoning, or mathematical skills

low potency homeopathic medicines—medicines of a 30C potency or lower

materia medica—a book containing individual homeopathic medicines and their indications for usage

miasm—an inherited or acquired layer of predisposition

mood stabilizer—a class of psychiatric medication used primarily to treat bipolar disorder

naturopathic physician—a physician who has graduated from a four-year naturopathic medical school and who treats the whole person based on the principle of the healing power of nature

neuroleptic—another term used for antipsychotics, a class of psychiatric medications used to treat thought disorders such as schizophrenia

neurotransmitter—a chemical substance, such as serotonin or dopamine, that transmits nerve impulses in the brain and nervous system, affecting thinking, behavior, sensory, and motor function

NIMH—National Institutes of Mental Health

NT—see neurotypical

neurotypical (NT)—neurologically typical or somebody without AS.

nonverbal learning disability (NLD or NVLD)—consisting of early speech and vocabulary development with impairment of abstract reasoning, coordination, and communication

nosode—a homeopathic medicine, such as *Lyssin, Medorrhinum, Tuberculinum, Syphilinum,* or *Carcinosin,* that is made from the product of disease

obsessive-compulsive disorder (OCD)—a diagnostic category that includes symptoms of obsessive thought patterns and ritualistic behaviors

oppositional-defiant disorder (ODD)—a pattern of negative and defiant behavior involving argumentativeness, resentment, vindictiveness, and abdication of personal responsibility

pervasive developmental disorder (PDD)—a generic term

referring to a group of disorders including autistic disorder, Asperger syndrome, Rett's disorder, fragile X syndrome, and childhood disintegrative disorder

PDD-NOS—pervasive developmental disorder not otherwise specified i.e., the general criteria for PDD are met, but the criteria for a specific PDD are not satisfied

perseveration—repetitive pattern of behavior or activity

phobia—an unreasonable, disproportionate, persistent fear of a specific thing

potency—the strength of a homeopathic medicine as determined by the number of serial dilutions and successions

prover—a person who takes a specific homeopathic substance as part of a specifically designed homeopathic experiment to test the action of medicines

provings—the process of testing homeopathic substances in a prescribed way in order to understand their potential curative action on patients

relapse—the return of symptoms when a homeopathic medicine is no longer acting

remedy—another word for a homeopathic medicine

repertory—a book that lists symptoms and the medicines known to have successfully treated those symptoms

return of old symptoms—the transient re-experiencing of symptoms from the past, after taking a homeopathic medicine, as part of the healing process

selective serotonin reuptake inhibitor (SSRI)—a class of antidepressant medications that increases serotonin levels in the brain

self-stimming—slang for repetitive behaviors such as twirling, hand-flapping, and flicking

sensory integration disorder—difficulty properly filtering sensory information so that the strength of a stimulus is misinterpreted

serotonin—a neurotransmitter in the brain which effects moods, sleep, and behavior

simillimum—the one homeopathic medicine that most clearly matches the symptoms of the patient and that produces the greatest benefit

state—an individual's stance in life; how he or she approaches, responds to, and experiences the world

stimulant—a substance, prescription or recreational, that heightens attention and alertness

succussion—the systematic and repeated shaking of a homeopathic medicine after each serial dilution

symptom picture—a constellation of all the mental, emotional, and physical symptoms that an individual patient experiences

theory of mind (TOM)—the capacity, which many with AS lack, to understand that other people have thoughts, feelings, motivations, and desires that are different from our own

thimerosal—a mercury-based preservative used in some vaccines

tic disorder—a condition characterized by twitches, jerks, and other compulsive or uncontrollable behaviors

totality—all of the symptoms of a patient, including physical, mental, and emotional

Tourette syndrome (TS)—a specific type of tic disorder that includes jerking, throat clearing, swearing, and other uncontrollable nervous system behaviors

vital force—the invisible energy present in all living things that creates harmony, balance, and health

Notes

1 Heinlein, RA. (1995). *Stranger in a Strange land: Remembering tomorrow*. (Reissue edition) New York: ACE Charter Publishing, p. 22-4

2 Heinlein, op. cit.

3 Interestingly, sometimes children with AS have a much easier time identifying "emotions" in a stick-figure type drawing than on a "real" face, either live or in a photograph. The stick-figures seem to reduce better to the kinds of "symbols" that AS kids often learn quickly and get comfortable with—a smile is a smile on a little stick man, whereas a smile on a person could be a mocking smile or a sad smile or a joyful smile, or all the degrees in between.

4 Twachtman-Cullen, D. (May-June 2004) Hyperlexia: A language treatment perspective. *Autism Asperger's Digest*, Future Horizons.

5 Zito, J.M. et al. (2003) Psychotropic practice patterns for youth: A 10-year perspective. *Archives of Pediatrics and Adolescent Medicine*, 157 (1), 17-25.

6 Ibid.

7 Ibid.

8 The National Institutes of Mental Health (NIMH) funds the Research Units of Pediatric Psychopharmacology (RUPP) network. The RUPP network is composed of research units that conduct studies which test the efficacy and safety of medications commonly used by practitioners to treat children and adolescents, but have not yet been adequately tested (off-label use).

9 Tsai, L.Y., (1999) Psychopharmacology in autism. *Psychosomatic Medicine*, 61, 651-665.

10 Harris, G. (2004, September 15) F.D.A. panel urges stronger warning on antidepressants. *New York Times,* p. A1.

11 Ibid.

12 Phelps, L., Brown, R., Power, T. (2002) Mental retardation and autistic spectrum disorders. In Phelps, L., Brown, R., Power, T. (Eds), *Pediatric psychopharmacology: Combining medical and psychosocial interventions.* (pp.146-161) NewYork, USA. American Psychological Association.

13 McCracken, J.T. et al. (2002) Risperidone in children with autism and serious behavioral problems. *New England Journal of Medicine,* 347 (5), 314-321.

14 Lansky, A. (2003). *Impossible cure: The promise of homeopathy.* California: R.L. Ranch Press.

15 Jacobs, J., Jimenez, L.M., Gloyd, S., Gale, J., Crothers, D., (1994) Treatment of acute childhood diarrhea with homeopathic medicine. *Pediatrics,* 93, 719-725.

16 Jacobs, J., Springer, D.A., and Crothers, D., (2001) Homeopathic treatment of acute otitis media in children: A preliminary randomized placebo-controlled trial. *Pediatric Infectious Disease Journal,* 20, 2, 177-183.

17 Linde, K., Clausius, N., Ramirez, G., Melchart, D., Eitel, F., Hedges, L., Jonas, W., (1997) Are the clinical effects of homeopathy placebo effects? A meta-analysis of placebo-controlled trials, *The Lancet,* 250, 834-843.

18 Kleijnen, J., Knipschild, P., ter Riet, G., (1991) Clinical trials of homeopathy. *British Medical Journal,* 302, 316-323.

19 California Department of Developmental Services. (1999) *Changes in the population of persons with autism and pervasive developmental disorders in system: 1987 thru 1998.* A report to the legislature March 1, 1999. California, USA: CDDS

20 California Department of Developmental Services. (2003). *Autistic spectrum disorders: Changes in the California caseload: an update; 1999-2002.* California, USA: CDDS.

21 California State Senate Committee on Health and Human Services. (2002) *Childhood Immunizations Mandates: Politics vs. Public Health.* California, USA

22 M.I.N.D. Institute. (2002) *News from UC Davis health*

system: Study confirms autism increase. California, USA: M.I.N.D. Institute.

23 Wing, L. & Gould, J. (1979). Severe impairments of social interaction and associated abnormalities in children: Epidemiology and classification. *Journal of Autism and Developmental Disorders,* 9 (1), 11-29.

24 Ehlers, S. & Gillberg, C. (1993) The epidemiology of Asperger's syndrome. A total population study. *Journal of Child Psychology and Psychiatry,* 34 (8), 1327-1350.

25 Chakrabarti, S. & Fombonne, E. (2001) Pervasive developmental disorders in preschool children. *Journal of the American Medical Association,* 285 (24), 3093-3099.

26 Scott, F.J., Baron-Cohen, S., Bolton, P., & Brayne, C. (2002) Brief report: Prevalence of autism spectrum conditions in children 5-11 years in Cambridgeshire, UK. *Autism,* 6 (3), 231-237.

27 Fombonne, E. (2003) Epidemiological surveys of autism and other pervasive developmental disorders: An update. *Journal of Autism and Developmental Disorders,* 33 (4): 365-382.

28 Bailey, A., Le Couteur, A., Gottesman, I., Bolton, P., Simonoff, E., Yuzda, E., Rutter, M. (1995) Autism as a strongly genetic disorder: Evidence from a British twin study. *Psychological Medicine,* 25 (1), 63-77.

29 Bolton, P., Macdonald, H., Pickles, A., Rios, P., Goode, S., Crowson, M., Bailey, A., Rutter, M. (1994) A case-control family history study of autism. *Journal of Child Psychology and Psychiatry,* 35(5), 877-900.

30 Geier M.R., & Geier D.A. (2003) Neurodevelopmental disorders after thimerosal-containing vaccines: A brief communication. Experimental Biology and Medicine, 228 (6) 660-664.

31 Centers for Disease Control. (1999) Notice to readers: Thimerosal in vaccines: A joint statement of the American Academy of Pediatrics and the Public Health Service. *MMWR Weekly,* 48(26), 563-565.

32 Chess, S. (1977) Follow up report on autism in congenital rubella.*Journal of Autism and Child Schizophrenia,* 7 (1), 69-81.

33 Deykin, E.Y. & MacMahon B. (1979) Viral exposure and autism. *American Journal of Epidemiology,* 109 (6), 628-638.
34 Ghaziuddin, M., Al-Khouri, I., Ghaziuddin, N. (2002) Autistic symptoms following herpes encephalitis. *European Journal of Child and Adolescent Psychiatry,* 11 (3), 142-146.
35 Lord, C., Mulloy, C., Weendelboe, M., & Schopler, E. (1991) Pre- and perinatal factors in high functioning females and males with autism. *Journal of Autism and Developmental Disorders,* 21 (2), 197-209.
36 Narita, N., Kato, M., Tazoe, M. Miyazaki, K., Narita, M., Okado, N. (2002) Increased monoamine concentration in the brain and blood of fetal thalidomide and valproic acid exposed rat: Putative animal models for autism. *Pediatric Research,* 52 (4), 576-579.
37 Davis, E., Fennoy, I., Laraque, D., Kanem, N., Brown, G., Mitchell, J. (1992) Autism and developmental abnormalities in children with perinatal cocaine exposure. *Journal of the National Medical Association,* 84 (4), 315-19.
38 Ghaziuddin, M., Weidmer-Mikhail, E., Ghaziuddin, N. (1998) Comorbidity of Asperger syndrome: A preliminary report. *Journal of Intellectual Disabilities Research.* 42 (Pt 4), 279-83.
39 Romanowski, P. & Kirby, L. (2001) *The oasis guide to Asperger syndrome: Advice, support, insight and inspiration,* New York, Crown Publishers, 69.
40 Ghaziuddin, M., Weidmer-Mikhail, E., Ghaziuddin, N. (1998) Comorbidity of Asperger syndrome: A preliminary report. *Journal of Intellectual Disabilities Research.* 42 (Pt 4), 279-83.
41 Tsai, L.Y., (1999) Psychopharmacology in autism. Psychosomatic Medicine, 61, 651-665.
42 Ehlers, S. & Gillberg, C. (1993) The epidemiology of Asperger's syndrome. A total population study. *Journal of Child Psychology and Psychiatry,* 34 (8), 1327-1350.
43 Tony & Temple: Face to Face, Jan-Feb 2000, *Autism Asperger's Digest,* Future Horizons
44 An Interview with Tony Attwood and Temple Grandin, *Autism Asperger's Digest,* Jan-Feb 2000, Future Horizons.

45 Romanowski, P. & Kirby, L. (2001) *The oasis guide to Asperger syndrome: Advice, support, insight and inspiration,* New York, Crown Publishers, 114

46 Baron-Cohen, S. (2000) Is HFA/AS necessarily a disability? *Development and Psychopathology.* January, 2000.

47 Frith, U. (2001) Asperger and his syndrome. In U. Frith (Ed.), *Autism and Asperger Syndrome* (pp. 1-36). Cambridge: Cambridge University Press.

48 Sacks, O. (1995) *An anthropologist on mars: Seven paradoxical tales.* New York: Alfred A. Knopf.

49 Wakefield, A.J., Puleston, J.M., Montgomery, S.M., Anthony, A., O'Leary, J.J. (2002) Review article: The concept of entero-colonic encephalopathy, autism and opioid receptor ligands. *Alimentary Pharmacological Therapy* 16: 663-74

50 D'eufemia, P., Celli, M., Finocchiaro, R., Pacifico, L., Viozzi, M., Zaccagnini, E., Cardi, E., Giardini, O. (1996) Abmormal intestinal permeability in children with autism. *Acta Paediatrica,* 85:1076-1079

51 Horvath, K., Herman, J.A. (2002) Autism and gastrointestinal symptoms. *Current Gastro-Enterological Reports,* 3:251-8.

52 Reichelt, K.L., Knivsberg, A.M. (2003) Can the pathophysiology of autism be explained by the nature of the discovered urine peptides? *Nutritional Neuroscience,* 6:19-28.

53 Whiteley, P., Shaddock, P. (2002) Biochemical aspects in autism spectrum disorders: Updating the opioid-excess theory and presenting new opportunities for biomedical intervention. *Expert Opinions of Therapeutic Targets,* 6: 175-83.

54 Thompson, T. (2003) Oats and the gluten-free diet. *Journal of the American Dietetic Association,* 103: 376-9

55 Gottshall, E. www.breakingtheviciouscycle.info.

56 Mattes, J.A., Gittelman, R. (1981) Effects of artificial food colorings in children with hyperactive symptoms: A critical review and results of a controlled study. *Archives of General Psychiatry,* 38: 714-8.

57 Rowe, K.S., (1988) Synthetic food colourings and 'hyperactivity': A double-blind crossover study. *Aust Paediatr J.* Apr; 24(2):143-7.

58 Rowe, K.S., Rowe, K.J., (1994) Synthetic food coloring and behavior: A dose response effect in a double-blind placebo-controlled repeated-measures study. *Journal of Pediatrics*, 125(5 Pt 1):691-8.

59 Feingold Association of the United States (2003) *Behavior, learning and health: The dietary connection.* New York: FAUS, 14.

60 Ibid. 14.

61 Ibid..

62 Rimland, R., (1987) Vitamin B6 (and magnesium) in the treatment of autism. *Autism Research Review International,* 1, no.4, 3.

63 Ibid.

64 Ibid.

Index

Homeopathic medicines appear in italics.

A

Abilify, 23
Academic ability, 108-109,
    113, 164, 179, 188, 202
Acute illness, 28, 32-33, 52,
    254, 264
ADD. *See* attention deficit
    disorder
ADHD. *See* attention-
    deficit/hyperactivity
    disorder
Adderall, 21, 76
Advice to parents of children
    with ASD, 240-246
    evaluating whether home-
        opathy can help,
        25-36
    discipline, 244
    joining, 245
    loving, 240
    managing your time,
        240-241
    proactive, 243-244
Aggravation, homeopathic,
    27, 44, 106, 251, 253,
    264
Aggression, 18, 95-96, 98,
116, 127, 165, 169, 175,
    177, 228, 237, 239
Allopathic medicine. *See*
    Conventional medicine
Allergies, *xxii*, 210, 219, 221-
    222, 256. *See also* Food
    Allergies
Aluminum, 223
American Academy of
    Pediatrics (AAP), 193
Amoxicillin, 104, 174, 177
Anger, 82-83, 85, 87, 123,
    160, 168, 227-231
Animal Planet, 90
Animals, relationship to,
    78-79, 82, 104, 108, 110,
    117, 136, 138, 139, 151,
    158, 161-165
Anti-anxiety medications,
    xvii
Antibiotics, 32, 106, 174
Anticonvulsants, *xvii*
Antidepressants, *xvii*, 22 32
Antidote, 51, 264
Anti-inflammatories, 32
Antimony, 212, 223
Anti-psychotics, *xvii*, 23-24,
    32

About the Authors

Judyth Reichenberg-Ullman, ND, DHANP, LCSW; Robert Ullman, ND, DHANP; and Ian Luepker, ND, DHANP are licensed naturopathic physicians and board-certified diplomates of the Homeopathic Academy of Naturopathic Physicians.

Dr. Reichenberg-Ullman received a doctorate in naturopathic medicine from Bastyr University in 1983 and a master's in psychiatric social work from the University of Washington in 1976. Dr. Ullman received his degree in naturopathic medicine from the National College of Naturopathic Medicine in 1981 and completed graduate coursework in psychology at Bucknell University in 1975. Dr. Luepker graduated *cum laude* from Connecticut College in 1992 with a degree in philosophy and received his ND from the National College of Naturopathic Medicine in 2002.

Dr. Reichenberg-Ullman and Dr. Ullman are former faculty members of Hahnemann College of Homeopathy and Bastyr University, and have presented seminars internationally. They co-authored seven other books including the best-selling *Ritalin-Free Kids*, as well as *Prozac Free, Rage-Free Kids, Homeopathic Self-Care,* and *The Patient's Guide to Homeopathic Medicine.* Dr. Reichenberg-Ullman also authored *Whole Woman Homeopathy.* Their 300-plus articles have appeared in many health publications, including a regular column in *The Townsend Letter for Doctors and Patients* since 1990. Dr. Reichenberg-Ullman has appeared on many radio shows including National Public Radio's *Talk of the Nation* and *Weekday*.

In practice for more than twenty years, Drs. Reichenberg-Ullman and Uilman have treated over 4,000 children with behavioral, learning or developmental problems. Dr. Luepker has been an associate in the practice since 2002, and has worked in both inpatient and outpatient mental health settings for over twelve years. The doctors practice at The Northwest Center for Homeopathic Medicine in Edmonds and Langley, Washington, where they specialize in homeopathic family medicine. In-person appointments, as well as telephone or videoconferencing consultations are available.

To contact their office, call (425) 774-5599 or visit www.drugfreeasperger.com. Their books can be ordered from Picnic Point Press, 131 3rd Ave, N., Edmonds, WA 98020; by calling (800) 398-1151; or online at www.healthyhomeopathy.com. For more information on Dr. Luepker, you can visit his website at www.sound-homeopathy.com.

To Order Books

Please send me the following items:

Quantity	Title	Unit Price	Total
_____	**Drug-Free Asperger**	**$22.95**	_____
_____	**Ritalin-Free Kids**	**$16.95**	_____
_____	**Rage-Free Kids**	**$19.95**	_____
_____	**Prozac-Free**	**$15.95**	_____
_____	**Homeopathic Self-Care**	**$19.95**	_____
_____	**Homeopathic Self-Care Book and Kit**	**$99.95**	_____
_____	**Whole Woman Homeopathy**	**$22.95**	_____
_____	**The Patient's Guide to Homeopathic Medicine**	**$12.00**	_____
_____	**Mystics, Masters, Saints and Sages**	**$16.95**	_____

Deduct 20% when ordering 5 or more books **Subtotal** _____

Shipping & Handling _____

- Order by phone with MC/Visa
  call: **1-800-398-1151**

Total Order _____

- Order online:
  www.healthyhomeopathy.com
- Order by email:
  ppp@healthyhomeopathy.com
- Order by mail: complete information
  below and send with remittance to:

Picnic Point Press
131 Third Avenue North
Edmonds, WA 98020

Shipping and Handling depend on Subtotal.

Subtotal	Shipping/Handling
$1.00-$24.99	$6.50
$25.00-$74.99	$8.50
$75.00-$149.99	$10.50
$150.00-$249.99	$14.50
$250.00-$399.99	$18.50
$400.00-$599.99	$22.50
$600.00+	Call for quote

Foreign and all Priority Request orders: Call us for price quote at 1-800-398-1151

Name_____

Address_____

City_____State_____ZIP_____

MC/Visa#_____Exp._____

Check/Money order enclosed for $_____ *Payable to Picnic Point Press*

Daytime telephone_____

Signature_____

Printed in the United Kingdom
by Lightning Source UK Ltd.
112251UKS00001B/110

9 780964 065468